D1118489

THE NUTS
AND BOLTS
OF LIFE

THE NUTS AND BOLTS OF LIFE

WILLEM KOLFF
AND THE INVENTION OF THE
KIDNEY MACHINE

PAUL HEINEY

SUTTON PUBLISHING

First published in 2002 by
Sutton Publishing Limited · Phoenix Mill
Thrupp · Stroud · Gloucestershire · GL5 2BU

This paperback edition first published in 2003

Copyright © Paul Heiney, 2002, 2003

All rights reserved. No part of this publication may be
reproduced, stored in a retrieval system, or transmitted, in
any form, or by any means, electronic, mechanical,
photocopying, recording or otherwise, without the prior
permission of the publisher and copyright holder.

Paul Heiney has asserted the moral right to be identified as
the author of this work.

British Library Cataloguing in Publication Data
A catalogue record for this book is available from the
British Library.

ISBN 0 7509 2896 4

Typeset in 11/13.5pt Sabon.
Typesetting and origination by
Sutton Publishing Limited.
Printed and bound in England by
J.H. Haynes & Co. Ltd, Sparkford.

CONTENTS

Acknowledgements   vii

Introduction   1

1   At Last, a Life Saved   9

2   Afraid to See People Die   17

3   Sausage Skin – an Unlikely Lifesaver   33

4   A New Mission – to Make People Sick!   52

5   Pots, Pans and a Splashing Machine   66

6   A Machine of Last Resort   88

7   A Miserable Convoy of Men and Boys   100

8   Peacetime Brings a Patient   113

9   Night Trains and New Ideas   121

10   The King of Kampen Loses his Crown   132

11   Replacing the Heart and Soul   155

12   'My Collaborators'   171

Appendix: Curriculum Vitae   181

Notes on Sources   183

Index   185

ACKNOWLEDGEMENTS

It is brave to entrust the story of your life to a complete stranger and I am grateful to Willem Kolff for having sufficient confidence to allow me to tell his remarkable tale. It has been not only a pleasure, but an inspiration to work with one of the greatest medical inventors of the twentieth century. He has been generous with his time, and patient. I could not have hoped to work alongside a more principled man.

My thanks to Jack and Adrie Kolff for the memories they have shared; and to Janke Kolff.

Jacob (Bob) van Noordwijk has been of enormous assistance to me. His detailed knowledge of events surrounding the early attempts at kidney dialysis is unmatched. He has generously allowed me to quote from his own book, *Dialysing for Life*, and has been a great help throughout this project. My thanks also to his wife Toos, for her kind hospitality.

The people of Kampen are justifiably proud of what Kolff achieved, and for the helpful spirit in which they approached this project I thank the Mayor of the city, also Dr John Jacobze of the Prof. W. Kolff Institute, and his wife Annette. Also my thanks to Herman Wessels of the Hotel Van Dijk.

I am fortunate to have had the assistance of J. Stewart Cameron CBE, MD, BSc, FRCP, Emeritus Professor of Renal Medicine at Guy's Hospital, London, and President of the International Society of Nephrology from 1993 to 1995. His recent history of dialysis (see Notes on Sources) must be considered the definitive work on this subject, and he has been generous in leading me carefully through a world hitherto unfamiliar to me, that of the workings of the kidney and the issues surrounding dialysis.

My thanks to the Ipswich hospital for allowing me to visit their dialysis unit, and in particular to Dr Paul Ford-Williams, Philip Lunts and Heather Moss, and the patients who spared time to share their experiences.

The transcription of many hours of tapes was done with great accuracy by Katherine Harvey. Due to his failing eyesight, the final manuscript of this book was read to Kolff by Diana Carroll, and my thanks to her. Also to the staff of the Wellcome Library of the History of Medicine.

For photographs, my thanks to Adrie Burnett, Bob van Noordwijk, Dr Sony Jacob, the Marriott Library and the Frans Walkatz Archief in Kampen.

Finally, my thanks go to Sutton Publishing for recognising that Kolff's story has appeal far beyond the bounds of the medical world.

Paul Heiney
Suffolk, 2003

INTRODUCTION

This story begins in Cornwall, in south-west England, where an old man of ninety is visiting his daughter. I am sitting with him on a wooden bench in the kitchen, eating breakfast, when the white-haired gentleman asks me to stand up because there is something he wants me to see.

Together we rise, then he stoops to pick up the bench, and turns it upside down in his hands. He flicks a catch, then another, and suddenly the legs have folded neatly away and what was a cumbersome piece of furniture has become no more than the plank of wood from which it was made. With the flourish of a magician, he does it again to prove to me that it works, even more delighted at his second performance than at the first. He turns to me, and although his eyes are failing I see them sparkle when he announces, 'I made it. I invented it.'

He is Willem Kolff, one of the greatest medical inventors of the modern age. He is no pharmacist, no surgeon; instead he has battled to mend broken bodies by bringing mechanical solutions to medical problems. He built the first ever artificial kidney and a working artificial heart, and helped create the artificial eye. He is the true founder of the bionic age in which all human parts will be replaceable. But in that kitchen, at that moment, the folding bench might have been the zenith of his lifetime's achievements, for after seventy years of inventing the thrill of the demonstration of the practical solution to the apparently insoluble problem has never dimmed.

To get a measure of his achievement, he suggested I checked in at my local hospital for a day, which I did.

He promised that if I turned up at virtually any hospital in the world on any day of the week, I would see people routinely being saved from death, thanks to his most famous invention.

I arrived at seven in the morning and followed the signs to the Kidney Unit. Like the organs themselves, which lurk around the back of the body, inconspicuously keeping us alive, kidney units are often at the rear of hospitals, taken for granted and expected to get on with their routine task, basking in little glory.

That morning the unit was bustling. The patients, if they were sick, didn't look it. If they were uncomfortably close to death's door, you would never have guessed. They looked like ordinary, healthy folk, just like you and me.

One was a truck driver who told me he wanted to be out by lunchtime to drive a load north. Another was a writer on a local newspaper who had a play to review that night. There was a shopkeeper who put the running of the business into his wife's hands for three mornings every week while he came here, and was happy to do so because he told me he didn't like most of his customers anyway and was glad to see the back of them. Ordinary people, ordinary lives. Only one thing set them apart – the day they don't show up here they are as good as dead.

Like members of a club, they knew each other. The pleasantries between them were brief, then with an air of resignation they lay back on reclining couches. Time spent here, they understood, was an intrusion into their lives which had to be endured, and they knew that impatience could not speed the process. This is a lesson some of them have learnt over years of visits to this clinic for never less than five hours at a time, three times a week. It is longer than some working people spend with their families: a huge chunk out of their lives.

INTRODUCTION

Like seasoned passengers on tedious long-haul flights, they knew all the tricks of making themselves comfortable. Some had even brought their own cushions with them; a few, who had mastered the art of reading and page turning with one hand immobilised while connected to the kidney machine, had brought a book. Some reached for the remote control which brought to life a television screen above each bed. It was well rehearsed and relaxed. Yet the cruel truth is that without the aid of the artificial kidney machine, with which the love/hate relationship can last for years, these and a million other people currently alive in the world would undoubtedly be dead. The patients I met that morning knew it. They understood that the vital cleansing effect of their own kidneys had failed them, and so that damned machine must do the work instead.

Over the years some learn to understand as much about the kidney machines as the nurses and technicians who operate them. They learn the settings that suit them best and can 'play' them for comfort as easily as setting the volume on a radio. But what they probably will not know is the remarkable story of how their saviour, the artificial kidney, was invented.

For the moment they will not care, for there is painful plumbing to be got over first. As carefully and as painlessly as she can, a nurse inserts a needle into an artery in their arm to connect the patient to the machine. The artificial kidney itself is a benign-looking creature, no more sinister than the marriage of washing machine and home computer. It is not for the squeamish, however, for the passage of crimson blood through it is clear to see, although kidney patients are seemingly used to the sight of their own blood, given that it is pumped repeatedly through a machine three times a week in their full view.

'Marvellous things, bottle tops', says Rosie, cheerfully. She is the patient who works on the local paper and says her visits here leave her feeling 'washed out! As though I've been through the wringer.' Washed out is, of course, a precise description of what is happening to her. The artificial kidney is washing her blood, ridding it of toxins that would kill her, poisons that will accumulate, causing other organs to falter. Yes, she will be washed out, but made fresh again to lead a normal life for a couple of days, and then she'll be back.

I asked her what she meant about 'bottle tops'. Proudly she rolled up her sleeve to reveal two white caps from juice bottles stuffed with white cream covering what looked like two heavy bruises on her arm. It was anaesthetic cream, to ease the pain when the needles were inserted. Not everyone bothered and grew used to the thrice-weekly stab. Rosie preferred to have the edge taken off it. This way she felt nothing.

'The doctor is happy to prescribe the cream, but he won't supply the bottle tops', she jokes as the nurse swiftly and deftly inserts the needle. She doesn't flinch. Instead, she rattles off instructions to the nurse as to how she'd like the machine adjusted, as casually as if she were describing to a hairdresser how hot she would like the dryer. 'Have you felt a fistula?' she offers, and reaches out her arm. She guides my hand and presses one of my fingers on to her wrist. Her wrist buzzes where a vein and artery have been surgically joined to provide a reusable connection to the machine. The buzz makes it feel as though she is full of electricity; indeed, what I am feeling is her life force, the surge of blood through her body.

I tell her I have recently met Willem Kolff, and that he was the doctor who, just over half a century ago, invented the machine which now stands beside her, contains much of her blood, and is making it pure again. I tell her that he is an old man now, turned ninety, but still bright of eye and with a brain people half his age would kill for. I remark that with his mop of pure white hair, beard and gentle smile, he could be mistaken for Father Christmas. She is mildly interested, but not ecstatic. And why should she be? You don't pause to think of the man who invented brake linings every time you put your foot on the pedal. No, some inventions have become too commonplace for that.

The artificial kidney has become such an accepted life support tool that it is difficult to imagine a time when it was not part of a physician's life-saving armoury. Yet without the groundbreaking events of fifty or so years ago, Rosie would not have been going to the theatre that night to pen her review, mothers would not be going home to feed their children, good lives would otherwise have been brought to a premature conclusion.

And not a pleasant end, either. The kidneys, a pair of organs no larger than a fist, are the body's public health department – there to ensure the blood is fresh and clean so that all the other organs of the body can go about their work without fear of infection or malfunction. Like a tidal barrier, they ensure that the body is awash with exactly the right amount of water, getting rid of excess as urine, and that in the remaining water the crucial balance between the vital elements potassium, sodium and calcium is maintained. But when the kidneys fail, like a city where the sewers won't work, the body starts to sink into a mire of its own waste. In a lecture on the 'Wonders of Medicine' given in 1937, a decade before real progress was made on the invention of the artificial kidney, Paul Lester Gronstein said, 'Even the greatest miracles we think we have achieved are patchwork. The true miracles are Nature's. One of the greatest is the kidney. But if you were to ask me how and why each of these curious "beans" is capable of performing such a tremendous amount of work, I would have to admit that I don't know. I know only this: the human being whose two kidneys are destroyed by malformations or diseases is hopelessly condemned to death. And we must look on helplessly.'

The kidney is a hugely complex filter consisting of microscopic tubes, the glomeruli, and if all of them were placed end to end they would cover a hundred miles. Just under 2,000 litres of blood are treated by our kidneys every day of our lives. Relentlessly they remove 1.5–2 litres of waste every day. Imagine if someone shut down the treatment plant, and the waste could make no escape. Nothing sudden would happen. Instead, as if standing in a slowly rising tide, you would become aware that you were being engulfed. Your blood pressure would soar, headaches may become unbearable, blindness might overtake you and eventually you would have convulsions. You would be suffering from uraemia: an accumulation of nitrogen-based wastes, measured by the level of urea in your bloodstream. Your body would seek every opportunity to rid itself of the urea, to the extent that crystals of it would try to force their way through your skin, and then the itching would drive you to mental distraction if your confused brain were still sufficiently active to recognise it. Then, without access to an artificial kidney machine, you would die.

A kidney transplant? If you are young and otherwise healthy, you might be lucky, despite a chronic world shortage of organs for transplant. Transplantation, without doubt, offers the best chance of long-term survival. Even so, the kidney machine remains a vital life support tool while you wait for your number to come up and a matching organ is found. However, if you are not one of the patients on what might be called a 'favoured' list, perhaps because you are older or have additional complications, then it is only the dialysis machine that keeps you from death's door. Not that a machine working outside the body, to which you have to be plugged in at regular intervals, could ever be considered better than a fully functioning kidney inside the body – patients who have been on dialysis and later been successfully transplanted will testify to that – but for people without the luxury of choice the kidney machine remains a life-saver.

As Rosie gets plugged in to her artificial kidney, she understands this all too well. She suffers from an inherited kidney disease that strikes in middle age. Her mother died of it. Her brother comes here three times a week, her thirty-year-old son is already showing symptoms and he too will soon be joining the early shift at the dialysis centre. 'They say that with a bit of luck I'll live to seventy or beyond. That's fine by me.' And while she closes her eyes for a few moments, the silent machine ensures that for another two or three days she will lead a near normal life. Then she'll be back for more.

When she woke, I decided to tell her the story of Willem Kolff and his invention, just as I'm going to tell it here. She ought to know how her life is being saved: we all ought to know that for a million of us, the throwing of the switch between life and death will be long delayed thanks to one inventive Dutch doctor who cheerfully admits, ' I sometimes wake up at four o'clock in the morning with an idea. And that's it! Problem solved.'

I wanted to tell her how I met the man who first brought together all the medical and engineering principles that make up the artificial kidney, and welded them into a machine which could make blood pure again. How, in wartime, in a small hospital in a town in the north-east of Holland, a medical miracle took place. How, with the oppressive Nazis breathing down his neck, Dr Kolff persisted with his ramshackle machine until, one groundbreaking night, he could look at his patient and know that for the first time an artificial organ working outside the body had saved a life. And that organ had been his invention. I wanted her to hear the story of how one man's unlikely blend of a medical and a mechanical mind could bring the world not only the artificial kidney, but eventually the heart/lung machine and even an artificial heart.

Kolff was eighty-nine when I first met him. If he faltered it was because his body was unable to match the speed of his brain. At the slightest prompting, he remembered every detail of the world's first artificial organ, the people who helped and hindered him, the places, the triumphs and the despair. I wish you could hear his voice for yourself. Although he speaks with the clarity of a scientist, choosing his words carefully, devoid of unnecessary emotion, his is the voice of a kind-hearted man. If you were sick, there could be no better voice to reassure you that everything would be well again. It is undeniably the voice of a Dutchman too; for although it is half a century since he left his homeland to live in the United States, there is little hint of America in his voice.

What follows is the story I told to Rosie during the five hours she lay plumbed in to her modern, state-of-the-art artificial kidney – a world away from Kolff's first machine of sixty years before, which was built out of wood and aluminium taken from a shot-down Nazi fighter plane, the parts welded together by a maker of pots and pans. It is the story which was told to me by Willem Kolff himself in detail he has never described before.

As I was about to leave, Rosie's doctor, the kidney specialist in charge of the unit, came up to me. He'd been watching Rosie and me in deep conversation and wanted to know what kind of story had electrified his normally torpid patient. I told him it was the story of Willem Kolff's invention of the artificial kidney.

His jaw dropped. He looked me in the eye and said, 'Kolff! You know Kolff? That man is God!'

I
AT LAST, A LIFE SAVED

What might a casual visitor have imagined was happening behind the closed door of Room 12a on the first floor of Kampen Hospital in a remote and rural corner of Holland on the night of 11 September 1945? There was little to suggest a small miracle was taking place; in fact, the sounds that emerged from that room could easily have been mistaken for an organised assault.

The sounds themselves were certainly sinister. There was a rumbling that echoed along the tiled corridors of the small hospital and kept patients on the floor below from their sleep; and the sound of what might be a paddle-steamer thrashing through water. All very curious.

And what of the people? Determined young girls dashed to the laboratory carrying urgent blood samples, and returned some hours later clutching the results which they scribbled in chalk on a board as if plotting the progress of some kind of military campaign. There was a young, tall doctor, with a long, thin face, who scrutinised the figures and appeared to be looking for any hopeful sign. He wore black-rimmed glasses, his hair was parted and combed back; he had the drawn look of a deeply tired man. The Second World War was over, and he had every right to be exhausted. He had risked his own life time after time to help rid his native Holland of the invaders, repeatedly stuck out his own neck to help the sick, protect his staff, conceal the oppressed Jews. Looking at him, it would come as no surprise to learn that he had taken to spending nights at the hospital, catching

9

a few moments' sleep on a stretcher. His own health had suffered and it showed in his thin frame. He drank only tea, or milky drinks prepared by the nurses, to soothe his stomach ulcer.

The 67-year-old patient lying in Room 12a would have been oblivious to all this. During the previous week she had suffered high fever, jaundice, inflammation of the gall bladder and kidney failure. Not quite comatose, she could just about respond to shouts or the deliberate infliction of pain. Her skin was pale yellow and the tiny amount of urine she produced was dark brown and cloudy. She had suffered like this for eight days, sleeping and snoring loudly all day, hardly stirring. When first admitted to the surgical ward on the 3rd, she had been partly lucid. But her mind became increasingly confused. Now, in order to communicate with her, the doctors would shout loudly in her ear, and in response she tried to utter a word or two from her parched throat. Her back and legs were swollen to hideous proportions. It was no kind of a life.

Death was common currency in the Netherlands at the end of the Second World War, no less for the war having just ended. Within recent weeks, some twenty thousand Dutchmen had died of hunger in a country on its knees at the end of a long fight. Some people were reduced to eating tulip bulbs as a last resort. Although the Netherlands had been liberated for five months, the struggle to feed the population in a country robbed of its food reserves by the Germans was as great as at any time during the war. Death was around them all the time, and they were weary of it.

Before she was wheeled into Room 12a of Kampen Hospital that night, Sofia Schafstadt's death was a foregone conclusion. There was no cure for her suffering; her kidneys were failing to cleanse her body of the waste it created in the chemical processes of keeping her alive. She was sinking into a body awash in her own poisons. By midnight her family had left her bedside, having prayed, one assumes, for a swift end to her suffering. They had been advised to say their goodbyes.

But that night was to be like no other night in medical history. The young doctor, Willem Kolff, then aged thirty-four and an internist at Kampen Hospital, brought to a great crescendo his work of much of the previous five years. That night, he connected Sofia Schafstadt to his artificial kidney – a machine born out of his own ingenuity. With it, he believed, for the first time ever he could replicate the function of one of the vital organs with a machine working outside the body. His assistants had prepared what, by modern standards, must have appeared to be a clumsy apparatus. They knew the routine. They boiled the glass and rubber connecting tubes to sterilise them, and washed them through with a drug, heparin, to prevent the blood clotting as it passed through. Then they took long lengths of cellophane tubing – an unlikely life-saving material, having originally been intended for use in the butchery trade as sausage skins – and started to wrap the tubing round and round the revolving drum at the heart of Kolff's apparatus. It must have looked as much like an artificial organ as a child's first attempts at Lego.

Sixteen times over the last three years Kolff had prepared what he believed would eventually be his life-saving machine. But fifteen patients had died. One had survived, but with no credit due to the kidney machine. If anyone thought the seventeenth experiment was similarly doomed to failure, they would never have spoken a word – they were too loyal to young Dr Kolff for that.

It was a hastily repaired machine which treated Sofia Schafstadt. Kolff's original, and so far unsuccessful, artificial kidney had been idle for almost a year while his hospital was awash with sick men and boys, the repatriated remnant of the tens of thousands of Dutchmen who had been rounded up and transported to Germany to work in Hitler's factories. In the great turning point of the war, on 6 June 1944, the Allies had landed in Normandy. Yet the Germans showed no intention of giving up the Netherlands without a fight to the very end. All but vital work at Kampen Hospital was abandoned as they prepared for the final battles of the war, which they doubtless expected to be the bloodiest. Kampen Hospital was no longer a place for medical experimentation or development. Its primary role was now as a front-line defence for the sick, injured and malnourished. So the experimental artificial kidney was pushed into a corner, where it was to become battered and damaged. Only after liberation could Kolff contemplate starting work again on his machine.

The machine itself was the size of a sideboard and stood by the patient's bed. The iron frame carried a large enamel tank containing fluid. Inside this rotated a drum around which was wrapped the unlikely sausage skin through which the patient's blood flowed. And that, in essence, was it: a machine that could undoubtedly be called a contraption was about to become the world's first successful artificial kidney. Nevertheless, as Kolff told me, 'There is nothing about the machine which someone with an elementary knowledge of science could not understand.' This is easy to say with hindsight, but the improbability of it at the time must have seemed overwhelming to those who didn't share Kolff's vision. The human kidney, although hugely complex in medical detail, fulfils a simple need. In the very process of living, of walking and breathing, even thinking, we burn energy which leaves behind waste, which is poisonous and must be got rid of. We dose our bodies too with all manner of 'foreign' chemicals, like pesticide residues, food additives and drugs, which must also be removed. The fluids in our body, the amount of water in them and the chemical balances within those solutions must also be kept within tight limits. The kidneys police all these things. When the natural kidney fails, the symptoms suffered by Sofia Schafstadt soon take over and death plays its trump card. The human kidney works by filtration. It allows the passage of unwanted chemicals through its membranes and into the urine while it retains the ones that are essential. Kolff, with his clanking apparatus and his sausage skin, was hoping to achieve the same effect. So far, after several years of experimentation, he had failed.

The patient was injected with heparin to prevent her blood clotting as it flowed through the machine. Then, on a nod from Kolff, a switch was thrown and the electrically driven drum began to spin at about twenty revolutions per minute. At first, Sofia Schafstadt went into uncontrollable shivering and hot water bottles were put into her bed to prevent the chill. These were merely the first steps on what was to be a long, hard road. Schafstadt was to lie connected to this machine for eleven-and-a-half hours. Although drawn and exhausted himself, Kolff never left her. Instead, he watched like a hawk the results being rushed from the laboratory across the corridor; the painstaking analyses were done through the night by his dedicated team of laboratory workers using classical methods of chemical analysis. Automated analysis was still a long way off.

The level of urea in the blood was what he watched most carefully, as this would give him an idea of how the dialysis was progressing. Urea is normally dealt with by the kidney and excreted with the urine. If Kolff could reduce the level of this and other life-threatening toxins in the blood with his machine, and restore the terminally ill patient to health, he would be able to claim that he had made the world's first artificial kidney machine, indeed the first ever artificial organ.

When Schafstadt was brought from the surgical ward to Room 12a where the artificial kidney had been set up, the level of urea in her blood was 4 grams per litre. The normal level is 0.45–0.5 grams per litre. She had no detectable kidney function. That was the size of Kolff's task, and for him there was no way to go but forwards. For Schafstadt, the only alternative was death.

For much of the eleven-and-a-half hours little appeared to have happened. Indeed, some of his workers remember the soporific effect of the constant rumble of the machine, and the regular splashing as the varnished wooden laths on the drum dipped in and out of the fluid bath. It was almost hypnotic in its rhythm.

Kolff and his staff were already tired, and the temptation to nod off must have been hard to resist. But vigilance was vital, for a tiny tear in the fragile sausage skin would allow the patient's blood to leak away and then the albumen in the seeping blood would be whipped into crimson foam by the revolving drum, in the same way that albumen in egg whites goes stiff under the action of the chef's whisk. Probably the most disturbing sight to confront a visitor to Room 12a on that night would have been the tiled floor awash in a sickly mixture of fluid and crimson foam. It didn't happen in every previous attempt at dialysis, but leaks could occur at any time. Sometimes wooden planks were laid down, supported on bricks, so Kolff and his nurses could walk around without soaking their feet. They would have preferred Wellington boots, but such luxuries were not available in post-war Holland.

After a while the machine was stopped and the tank of fluid into which the patient's toxins were being washed was changed for fresh. Then the rumbling started again.

After eleven hours her blood pressure had fallen to a normal level, and the urea was down from 4 to 1.2 grams per litre. Kolff switched off the machine. But despite the analytical evidence that his machine was indeed cleansing the blood, I doubt whether he paused to allow himself any self-congratulation. Exhausted, Kolff shunned an opportunity to go home to rest and instead stayed with his patient, anxious to answer the question which was uppermost in his mind – was this the breakthrough for which he had been longing, or was it yet another false dawn for his kidney machine?

Then Sofia Schafstadt awoke. Kolff spoke to her, and asked her how she was doing. Her reply was the product, one assumes, of profound thought through the depths of her terminal illness. In a low but strong voice, she turned to the man who had brought her back from the brink of death and said, 'Now I'm going to divorce my husband!'

And the irony was that Sofia Schafstadt had been a Nazi sympathiser; a true enemy of everyone who had worked with Kolff in that hospital through the gruelling war years. She had collaborated with the Germans for four years, and after the liberation had been sentenced to imprisonment by the Dutch authorities for her treachery. Much of the suffering that Kolff and his team had treated through the war years had been caused by the actions of traitors like Sofia Schafstadt. Kampen Hospital had treated the under-nourished, the shot and the maimed; the whole of the Netherlands had experienced bereavement on an unprecedented scale. They hated the Nazis and reviled traitors like Sofia Schafstadt.

Kolff too could have been excused any antipathy towards the woman. But as a doctor with a broad streak of humanity running through him, it would never occur to him that a patient might be treated differently from any other because of who they were or what they had done. He knew his ethical obligations.

Sofia Schafstadt was still in hospital under Kolff's care in early December, three months after her treatment on his kidney machine. It was St Nicholas's Eve, a day traditionally celebrated with gifts in the Netherlands. Schafstadt remembered, 'I was very sad. Everyone received presents except me.'

Only one person noticed her loneliness. And so who should appear round the corner of the ward, dressed as St Nicholas, bearing a gift for his traitorous patient? It was Dr Willem Kolff.

2
AFRAID TO SEE PEOPLE DIE

If anyone was going to have an instinctive understanding of the way fluids behave, how they can be controlled, a balance achieved, an inundation prevented, it was always going to be a Dutchman. The Dutch live in closer proximity to water than any other Europeans and it defines their country. At every turn they are confronted with water as it flows, at their behest, through canal and sluice and behind dykes. So at ease are they with it that many live, unconcerned, several metres below the level of the sea, protected by human engineering on a grand scale. Yes, the Dutch know how to engineer water to work for them, and not against them.

The Kolff family had water on all four sides. The village of Middelharnis, where Willem Kolff's grandfather Cornelius managed the area's most influential business, sits on what was once an island in the intricate delta formed where the rivers Rhine, Schelde, Waal and Maas spread their fingers and flow into the North Sea. Given its position close to not only the sea but also the entrance to the waterways that provide direct access to the heart of both the Netherlands and Germany, it is no surprise that nineteenth-century Middelharnis was a bustling village with shipyards and chandlers, as well as agricultural businesses serving the needs of the fertile island and hinterland. On an island, called Overflakkee, a comfortably well-off Cornelius Kolff acted as a land agent for farms and estates and ran several businesses of his own, even though he was unqualified in some areas.

Willem Kolff remembers his great aunt having a wine business although she apparently knew very little about wine. However, his grandfather was already a wealthy and influential man and a ship owner with a fleet of twelve fishing boats, each with a crew of twelve men, which fished on the Dogger Bank in the North Sea. Every New Year's Day the skippers of the boats would come and pay their respects in the morning, when a pile of large silver coins was waiting on the chimney mantle. Each of the twelve skippers would receive one.

Kolff remembers his grandfather waiting anxiously for his ships to come home. 'On top of one of his buildings was a small dome to which he would climb, and with an old-fashioned, very long looking glass, he would spy the horizon.' But on the occasions when the ships did not return, Kolff the ship owner did his duty by the village. 'He would don his black suit, put on his top hat, and stride slowly through the village, going from house to house to bring the bad news. The family of the crew would sit and wait, and pray to the good Lord that he would pass their house.'

Willem Kolff was born into what were still feudal times in the Netherlands, although a strong social conscience was evident in his family. When a ship returned from sea with a large amount of fish, some of the catch was cooked by Kolff's grandmother and given to a long list of needy people. Kolff remembers that, 'on one occasion when my grandmother was in Rotterdam, the oldest daughter, Em, took over the cooking of the fish and saw that the proper pans were delivered to the proper recipients. The following day, when the empty pans were returned, there was a message with one of them that said "Thank you very much. Does the young lady know that lemon goes with the fish?" This was to remind the oldest daughter that she had forgotten the lemon. It was meant as a joke by a grateful recipient of much-needed food.'

Grandfather Cornelius had seven children, and Jacob, the youngest, was Willem Kolff's father. It was at this stage in Kolff family history that two important traits were lost. First, all the sons deserted the fishing trade (Jacob gave it a brief go but it was not a great success for he was seasick most of the time). Secondly, the family's entrepreneurial flair seemed to evaporate too, or at least missed a beat somewhere in passing from Cornelius to Jacob and then to Willem. Towards the end of his career, Willem Kolff was to admit, with regret, that he was 'a good businessmen on other people's behalf, but not for myself'.

The Kolff family took a new direction when Jacob finally announced that he was never going to sea again (having failed to cure his seasickness by his father's recommended treatment of raw fish eaten off the hand), and instead intended to study medicine. He was drawn to the University of Leiden, the oldest in the Netherlands, which was founded in 1575 as a reward for the endurance of the population under siege by Spanish troops. Leiden is also the birthplace of Rembrandt, and the place where Clusius brought the first Dutch tulip into flower: an act as fundamental to the future identity of the Netherlands as the landing of the Pilgrim Fathers was to America.

For anyone wishing to study medicine, as Jacob Kolff did, the medical faculty at the city's classical university must have been an inspirational place, for here a young and impressionable student could imagine that the ghost of the medical giant Herman Boerhaave still walked. Described as the 'first great clinician', Boerhaave taught medicine at Leiden in the late seventeenth and early eighteenth centuries, becoming professor of botany and medicine, rector of the university and professor of both practical medicine and chemistry. In acts of pilgrimage, students travelled from all parts of Europe to hear him teach, and were greatly influenced by his then radical belief that the best place for learning and understanding medicine was at the patient's bedside.

Boerhaave's idea of medical learning and understanding was a simple one, and to demonstrate it he formed an association with a nearby hospital to which he regularly took groups of students. He chose a modest, twelve-bed ward to demonstrate his theories, which he did by standing beside each bed in turn, observing the patient, describing the symptoms, and teaching on the basis of what could be observed. It has since become known as the 'bedside manner', and, taken in conjunction with his stated belief that 'the conjunct power of all these actions of the body for preserving its own health, which arises from the wonderful structure of its parts, is what Hippocrates calls nature', it formed the basis of an entirely new, and still surviving, view of medicine which had until then been a detached, academic science. Yet for all Boerhaave's vision, it would have been beyond his belief that 150 years after his death the function of some of the body's parts would be maintained by a mechanical device, defying the will of nature itself, and that this extraordinary machine would be built by Willem Kolff, a student of Leiden University following in the Boerhaave tradition of defining new limits of medical discovery.

It was while Jacob Kolff was at Leiden, immersing himself in the inspirational atmosphere of the medical school, that he met the woman who was to become Willem Kolff's mother. They became engaged at a very early age, which was frowned upon. Kolff remembers, 'It was decided that my father and mother were allowed to meet each other one day per month and no more! I've seen letters from the father of the bride and my grandfather's letters in which they both regretted having to write to each other about their children's plans at such an early date.'

In what was to be an uncanny foretaste of the way Willem Kolff's supportive married life was to be played out, his mother decided that it was her duty to support Kolff's father in whatever way she could. She trained in a pharmacy in Rotterdam so that she could later assist in making medicines, since it was usual for doctors to have pharmacies in their own homes. After no fewer than seven years of engagement, they married and lived in the Hotel Rijnland. This may seem a strange place in which to begin married life, but the hotel was by the cattle market in Leiden, one of the biggest in the Netherlands, and was only two minutes' walk from the university hospital: 'My father had become an assistant in obstetrics and he could marry only on condition that he would live two minutes' walk from the university hospital to be available at all times when a child was going to be delivered.'

For that reason Willem Johann Kolff, nicknamed 'Pim', was born in a hotel room on 14 February 1911, in a hotel that smelt strongly of cattle dung. Kolff remembers, 'the cattle manure on the boots of the farmers and dealers invaded every corner of the Hotel Rijnland and made the floor of the lobby entirely green. And at the end of every market day, the floor was washed and restored to cleanliness, until next market day when it became indistinguishable again from the cattle pens outside.'

Hotel life was not to last for long. Jacob Kolff gave up his assistantship in obstetrics in Leiden, and in 1916 went to run a small general practice in a little village called Hummelo in the east of the Netherlands. To young Willem's eyes, this 'seemed to me to be the most beautiful, rural, part of the Netherlands'. He remembers the sounds, if not the sights, of the First World War. The Netherlands were never occupied by the Germans, but neighbouring Belgium was, and one of Kolff's earliest memories is of 'very heavy guns firing, the sound coming all the way across the border from Belgium itself. I remember seeing wagon loads of potatoes being hauled through the streets bound for Germany.'

From a professional point of view, Jacob Kolff's move to village practice was a great success, and provided an opportunity for the first doctor in the Kolff family to display the inventive talents of a very able physician. 'A man was splitting a metal band on an anvil. He was going to use it to reinforce his wooden shoe, or clog. It jumped up and punctured his neck just under his Adam's apple. All my father could see was a little metal tip sticking out of this man's neck, he had no idea what was in there, and neither did the man. My father grabbed the end and carefully began to pull. Unbelievably, a foot of metal came out. And the man had no further trouble after that. That's how skilful a physician my father was.'

There was never a quiet moment in a remote rural practice, and Kolff's father soon became ill with the stress of it, and went to Amsterdam for a surgical exploration of abdominal pains. 'They thought it might be kidney stones but they found nothing and sewed him back up. From then on, I think, the practice got too much for him. He spent a lot of time travelling from patient to patient on his motorcycle, sometimes with my mother riding in the sidecar, and it was heavy work. It was time for him to move on.'

The Netherlands is not a large country, and any move need not necessarily involve great distances, although the change in lifestyle for the Kolff family must have been enormous when Jacob gave up his rural practice to take up the directorship of a tuberculosis sanatorium in Beekbergen, south of Apeldoorn.

'It was in the sandy part of the Netherlands, which made it dry where the land was exposed to wind, and you had sand dunes like the Sahara. We went to the village school where everyone had wooden shoes, except my brother Kees and I who had leather shoes because we came from a better-off family.' Willem Kolff was now six years old.

Two seeds were planted in young Willem Kolff's impressionable mind during his father's stewardship of the Beekbergen sanatorium, and both led him indirectly towards his kidney machine and his artificial heart. The first inspiration was innocently provided by the sanatorium's carpenter, who taught young Pim how wood was cut, planed, screwed and joined, how it could be shaped and how figments of the imagination could be transformed into useful reality by the application of craft. This was a lesson Pim relished, with the result that Jacob did a deal with the carpenter, whereby he would teach Pim the carpenter's craft. He proved to be an impatient student. 'The carpenter warned me that there would not be something to take away after every Saturday afternoon session – some things took longer that that.' Some of the skills Willem learnt then he retains. He can still operate a chisel with his shoulder, leaning on it and guiding it to make the most precise of cuts. 'You don't use a hammer, just apply pressure from your body. You can cut very precisely that way. And, of course, you have both hands free.' Workshop days were the best of times for him. When he had mastered sufficient skills to make a simple wooden box, he sang all the way home. 'I was so overjoyed, clutching that little box. I had never been so happy.'

The idea of *making* something is very much part of Kolff. Given a choice, he will use wood and not metal 'which makes your hands dirty'. He admits to enjoying 'playing with water too' and to 'a natural understanding of hydrodynamics from a very early age, even if I didn't know what the word meant'. Those passions were to come together in later life, and would lead directly to his medical breakthrough. 'An understanding of simple hydrodynamics and physics is enough to build a kidney machine. You don't need to know any more that that.' Indeed, his first kidney machine was built on a *wooden* frame.

As influential as the hours spent knee-deep in wood shavings in the carpenter's shop were the sights which confronted him on a daily basis – the tuberculosis patients in his father's care. In 1920 there was still no cure for tuberculosis. That did not mean that everyone infected with it died from it, and Kolff himself, who bears a scar on his own right lung, is testament to the fact that tuberculosis *can* heal itself. In some cases fresh air was a tried and tested cure, but for patients with severe infections the treatments were harsh, debilitating and often deforming. The cause of the disease was known: it was the bacillus *Mycobacterium tuberculosis*, discovered by the German pathologist Robert Koch, the 'father of bacteriology'. That it might ever be cured by the administration of a drug was then beyond imagination if not hope. It was not until the discovery of streptomycin in 1943 (in the same period that Willem Kolff was developing his artificial kidney) that there came a final cure and a programme of worldwide eradication could begin. This was far beyond the lifespan of the patients Jacob Kolff treated in his Beekbergen sanatorium, for whom a certain cure lay some thirty years in the future. Consequently the treatments at Beekbergen were the same primitive 'cures' as were used the world over, often employed more in hope than expectation, The most benign was cold, fresh air in large quantities; this was thought to ease the condition, and in some cases it did.

Surrounded by the sick, Willem Kolff, at the impressionable

age of six, was confronted with the concept of mortality and didn't like what he saw. 'The first year we lived there, I was so afraid of seeing patients die.' He remembers the gruesome treatments his father attempted in extreme cases, such as giving pneumothorax to cause the lungs to collapse, or cutting the phrenic nerve so that the diaphragm wouldn't move any more. Sometimes he might take out ribs to collapse the whole lung on one side. Kolff remembers seeing several patients who had had that done to them. 'You could insert a large ball of paraffin between the ribs and the pleura, the covering of the lungs, and this would specifically compress and put out of action any part of the lung that was infected. Some of these patients my father had for twenty years and sometimes they still got well.'

Even so, to a six-year-old it must have seemed like a living death for many of these patients as they underwent disfiguring surgery, painful and uncertain procedures performed against a background of cacophonous coughing from those patients who had tuberculosis of the lungs. Willem Kolff, 'afraid to see patients die', wanted none of this for a career, and insisted instead that he wanted to be a zoo keeper. He kept pheasants, rabbits, a sheep, magpies and two parakeets, a mouse, a baby crow and a jackdaw. 'My dream was to have a real menagerie and I set out to build it when I was very young, and worked on it until I went to the University of Leiden to study medicine. I loved the magpies most.' They were less welcome, however, in the sanatorium, where usually there was a thermometer in a beaker standing on the night table. The magpies' sport was to remove all the thermometers from the beakers and drop them on the table. 'My magpies also liked to pick at the legs of my youngest brother just above his socks, which he didn't like at all. And the magpie would sit on your shoulder and there was always the chance that it would take your earlobe and twist it. Very painful! One day I noticed the feathers of the magpie all along the garden path. I followed the feathers and about twenty yards away I found the magpie dead. What killed it I never found out. I was very sad.'

For a lad smitten with the idea of becoming a zoo keeper, there was bad news on the way. His father gently pointed out that the Netherlands only had two zoos, one in Amsterdam and the other in Rotterdam, and the chances of becoming director of either were slim. At the age of eight, Willem bravely resigned himself to pursuing another career. The idea that he might become a doctor was slow to emerge. 'The reason I didn't want anything to do with medicine when I was very young was because I was afraid I would see a patient die. It's remarkable, isn't it,' he reflects, 'how the rest of my life has been devoted to patients who seemed certain to die, yet trying so hard to prevent them.'

The inspiration of watching his father's patient and meticulous care of the sick – a compassion that the young Kolff undoubtedly inherited – gave him the courage to overcome his self-doubt. 'My father had intense concern for his patients. Not just their medical case but their whole person. He didn't expect me to follow him as a doctor, he didn't push it. But it slowly became very clear that's what I wanted to do. I saw his work and how much he loved it, how much he was involved, and I wanted it.' On leaving school, he was soon following in the medical footsteps of his father. Pim Kolff went up to the University of Leiden in 1931. He remembers no discussion about his choice of medical school: 'It was just assumed I would go where my father went.'

Meanwhile, other feelings blossomed alongside his desire to be a doctor. Still a schoolboy, what he craved almost as much as a medical career was an 'elegant and thoughtful' girl called Pop van West, on whom he'd first set eyes at the age of seventeen. Life was very formal then, even more so for youngsters, and 'introductions' were required. Kolff engineered a suitable meeting, inviting a mutual friend to come and play tennis in the hope that Pop would come too. In passing, the friend suggested that he might also bring along his sister Janke, the girl Kolff would eventually marry.

Janke Huidekoper came from a very different family background. On her own admission she was 'a tomboy. My life was full of music, dancing, singing, card games and laughter. I didn't want any boyfriends in my life, especially those who were silly enough to show it openly!' Janke was strong and pretty, and according to friends Kolff pursued her like a creature possessed, admitting 'she was a hard nut to crack! And stubborn too.' Janke herself often spoke to her friends of her memories of the young Pim Kolff, describing him as 'too serious and too stiff'. His school was one-and-a-half blocks away from hers, but for chemistry and physics they had the same teachers. Between lessons, they sometimes met: 'He would meticulously take off his hat, which was an enormous embarrassment to me.' Later, in her schoolwork, she wrote in several places the letters P.K., which meant, in physics, 'paarde kracht' (horse power). What it really stood for, from her point of view, was Pim Kolff. But she did not make life easy for her suitor. One day, after school, she noticed him on his bike, holding on to a lamp post, obviously waiting for her. Furiously she jumped on her bike and pedalled home like a madwoman, leaving Pim far behind her and taunting him every inch of the way home.

Kolff remembers their five-year engagement, longing impatiently for marriage. 'We owned a small car; the first was an old DKW with a two-cylinder engine where you mix the oil and the gasoline, and the body was made of thin plywood and water had got in and it had rotted. When you opened the doors the hinges didn't work.' For a man to whom invention was second nature, this small problem with the motor car caused him no difficulty. He sorted it by drilling holes to hold a metal bar under the dashboard, and by tightening the nuts the sides of the car came together. 'We paid a total of fifty guilders for that automobile – at that time the equivalent of twenty dollars. It had an open roof and when you closed it with the canvas, the rain came through with such force that we usually looked for a big tree for shelter until the rain was over. Whenever the car behaved well we gave it a reward, and the first reward was a new roof.'

The late 1920s and early 1930s were depressed years in the Netherlands, as in much of Europe, but no compromises seem to have been made at the University of Leiden, certainly not among the better-off male students. 'The amazing thing was that the student life continued on the same footing as before. We were drinking champagne, and not the cheap stuff either, but Moët et Chandon or Veuve Clicquot. When you think back to it, it was ridiculous.'

Student life at Leiden was run on a feudal system, long after other seats of learning had relinquished such indulgence. It was ritualistic, often humiliating, with students having to endure a 'green' period before beginning their studies. Not everybody could stand it. 'Your hair was shaved, you had to sit on the floor for three weeks and were generally abused. You were treated like a dog. If you could get through that, and quite a few couldn't stand it, then you were admitted. I recall that I saw another "green" student sitting on the floor with a spoonful of mustard on his bald head, the mustard slowly dripping down his face. I wouldn't have taken that.'

The drunken student life was not to Kolff's liking. 'It was all right for law students who never made early starts – their lectures started at eleven. But for medical students the first lecture was at nine sharp. I remember that some mornings I was so tired that I rode my bicycle, half asleep, through the streets, and the street organs were just beginning to play, the sounds echoing round the empty medieval streets, and I navigated by the sound of the nearest street organ.'

The feudal system extended far beyond the ritualistic initiation of the students, and the more privileged students were given the services of an Oppasser, a sort of manservant who would come and polish your shoes or pack your suitcases if you had to travel, and brought tea in the morning. 'My father had an Oppasser too, and on my first day there the same man, Jan Sierat, came to see me and said, "I have been your father's Oppasser, I would like to take care of you too." Of course I accepted. We lived to a standard that was ridiculously high. Remember, this was in the depression years too.'

While Willem Kolff learnt medicine, Janke studied also. With her father's encouragement, she trained as a medical technician in Leiden, where she lived for three years. But when Janke was only eighteen her mother died from blood poisoning at the young age of forty-five. 'My whole life collapsed and I was suddenly not a child any more, I was a grown-up.' Four months later her grandmother died and Janke suddenly found herself a wealthy young woman. Her grandmother had inherited stock in a tropical quinine plantation, founded in the nineteenth century. With quinine still the only effective treatment against malaria, the stock paid huge dividends. 'My father gave me good advice,' Janke remembers, 'but I never had plans anyway to go into high society.' Instead, carefully preserving her capital, she spent the income on table silver and linen so that when she was married and had a home of her own, it would measure up to the standards of her childhood. She remembers it as being 'quite a trousseau'.

After finishing her studies Janke moved to a hospital in Alkmaar, north of Amsterdam, living in a small, white-painted room at the top of the hospital. The terms included free room and board, but the provisions were basic, consisting often of an egg, bread, and buttermilk porridge for pudding. Janke hated it, saying it turned her hair green. 'I quickly adjusted to that hard, simple life, scrubbing the floors of the laboratory on a Friday like all the other nurses.'

For social reasons a formal engagement was becoming a pressing matter for Pim's parents. The Netherlands before the Second World War was not a place where a girl could be seen in public on a young man's arm for too long. The female patients at Kolff's father's sanatorium, where Pim and Janke spent occasional weekends, repeatedly asked who the young woman was that they saw so often in Pim's company, and why had she not been introduced to them? They asked, pointedly, if a wedding date would soon be announced? But marriage was out of the question, for Janke had no desire for an early marriage and Kolff was still a mere student, and young men did not marry until they could support a wife. To add to his complications, a bizarre rule at Leiden said that residents who wished to specialise in internal medicine were not allowed to be married at all! It was argued that such young doctors needed to be available twenty-four hours a day and a wife might hinder a student's wholehearted concentration. One university, however, waived the rule – Groningen. Kolff made careful note of that for future use.

Even as a second-year student at Leiden, Kolff's inventive talents and capacity for original thought were becoming recognised. He became an assistant to the professor of pathology, the old but distinguished Tendeloo, who by then was a little senile. According to Kolff, he was 'past his prime, and extremely deaf. He said to me once, "Kolff, why are you out of breath?" I was, of course, breathless from shouting at him. But some of his genius remained and he was a very good teacher.'

Professor Tendeloo's budget stretched to only two full-time assistants, but in order to include Kolff in that number he engineered the appointment of three students and paid them less than the full wage. Despite the cut-price wages, the experience of working close to Tendeloo was a bargain in Kolff's eyes, for he was able to follow clinical cases and practise bedside medicine while learning Tendeloo's methods of clinical examination, diagnosis and treatment. Classes other than clinical ones, such as the more theoretical pharmacology, fell outside these privileges. Kolff remembers, 'I never learned pharmacology well and never liked it. I hired a tutor who could teach me enough to get me through the exam!'

But the experience of close contact with pathological anatomy more than made up for any deficiencies there might have been in his theoretical medical knowledge and provided him with an education that was to last a lifetime. 'During later years, when I saw a disease I could see the pathological, anatomical basis forming, and I didn't only see the macroscopic features of the disease but also the microscopic ones. Later when I went to work in the city of Kampen, I did autopsies on all patients that died. Some of my friends said I was in a "win/win situation" because you either cured the patient or you got them in the end anyway when they died. But in reality, this understanding of pathology was a great help and it was always a consolation when I found that the patient that I had lost had a disease that I could not possibly have cured.'

The study of medicine took seven years, during which time Kolff published his first scientific paper. It was a study of a rare skin disease, *Mycosis Fungoides*, inspired by an unusual case which Kolff discovered occurring in the intestines of a patient. 'A friendly professor of anatomy in Amsterdam sent me the data on a couple of cases he had seen and I published a few papers about it.'

He graduated from Leiden in 1938, and began to search for a job where he could qualify for his desired certificate as a specialist in internal medicine. Also in his mind was an overwhelming desire to marry his beloved Janke, and consequently there was only one university to which he made an application – Groningen. The promise of a position there would be a huge leap forward in his career. Indeed, of all the things Groningen was to give him, this might be considered just one of its great gifts.

3

SAUSAGE SKIN –
AN UNLIKELY LIFE-SAVER

With the promise of a position at Groningen secured, Kolff could marry at last. Six months before his graduation, he and Janke were wed on 4 September 1937 and settled in Noordweg, a resort on the North Sea coast. From here Kolff commuted daily to his studies in a borrowed and fondly remembered, if unreliable, blue Essex two-seater, leaving his new wife behind. The unexpected loneliness came as a shock to her. The house in which they lived, in a town which was effectively closed and isolated in the winter season, was of necessity cheap. Day in, day out she saw only a baker or a fishmonger. It was a bleak awakening.

Janke had taken her marital duties seriously and had attended a school at The Hague where young women were taught to be efficient wives by undergoing an education apparently based on unquestioned service to their husbands' every need. Janke learnt sewing, washing, cooking and ironing, and 'proper cleaning of the toilet'. Janke's education in the domestic arts provided the working basis of what these days would be considered an old-fashioned and dutiful marriage, of which Kolff said he never had any cause to complain. It was, in many ways, a nineteenth-century kind of arrangement which suited a man who had enjoyed a nineteenth century style of education and upbringing and found no fault with it. According to friends, Janke said in later years, with some resentment, that, 'Pim could always work wherever he was, providing the children were not arguing. That he could not take. So I suppose by keeping them out of his way so he could get on with his work, I was making my own contribution to science.'

In order to finish his degree, Kolff commuted daily to Leiden for six months, travelling in their stuttering old car. When his studies allowed, they walked the lonely, windswept winter beaches hand in hand: 'Sometimes the wind was so strong you could lean against it.' He finally took his degree in February 1938. The long winter interlude in Noordweg was over and at last Groningen beckoned.

Money was the first hurdle they had to overcome. Kolff knew well that the University of Groningen was, and remains, one of the major seats of learning in the Netherlands, and that it was the country's second oldest university, founded in 1614. Medicine was one of its original faculties. He was proud to be there but none of this kudos paid the bills. He was to be an assistant, an unpaid position with no prospect of a proper salary for four years. With the days of cheap living by the North Sea gone, somehow the rent had to be paid on the hotel room, which was their first home. Later they found a tiny first-floor apartment where they finally settled on the east side of the town, with a view over the Groningen countryside. Janke was also pregnant. A surge in the quinine market was to be their saviour. The shares Janke had inherited from her grandmother continued to pay a handsome dividend and provided their income throughout the Groningen days. Their first child, Jack, was born on 23 August 1938. This called for more than just the level head required of any new father. Jack recalls: 'Dad delivered me himself, and shortly after I was admitted to hospital for pyloric stenosis. When he needed to give me a transfusion, it was of his own blood.'

Married at last, and now a family man studying at Groningen University, Kolff could allow his mind to relax into medicine. Soon after Jack was born, his first ever invention was created in an academic atmosphere that clearly inspired him. He could have had no better tutor than Professor Polak Daniels, a Jew of great good humour, who was head of the internal medicine department at the university. A heavy man, thick necked, with a domed, bald head, Daniels took what was then the unusual step of encouraging his assistants in their private researches. Where other academics saw such research as an interruption to their own work, Daniels allowed those who worked under him to pursue their own ideas, make their own discoveries and publish them. Daniels was not the best-known professor of medicine in the Netherlands, but, as Kolff later observed, 'those who rose high in the medical profession were often his students'. For someone like young Kolff, with an inventive mind and a keenness to learn, there could hardly have been a richer atmosphere in which to work.

Kolff's very first application of a mechanical solution to solve a medical problem happened in Daniels's department. A patient with poor circulation in his legs needed urgent help to improve the flow of blood through the limbs. Kolff had seen a paper, published in the United States, which suggested the condition could be eased by 'intermittent occlusion of the venous return of the blood'. In other words, Kolff reasoned, if some way could be found of applying pressure to the legs to interrupt the flow of blood, and then releasing it to allow the blood to surge forward, he might be able to help this patient. If Kolff's career in medical invention began anywhere, it was here beside this patient's bedside, as he tried to conjure up in his mind some kind of mechanical device which would perform that seemingly simple task of squeezing the leg and then letting it go. Where other doctors might have contemplated a new surgical technique, or a pharmacist a drug, Kolff went back to his childhood, to the Saturday afternoons spent with the carpenter making boxes. He thought of tubes, wood, screws and water. He remembers: 'I built a little apparatus which would be connected with a water tap at one end, and that water filled a series of reservoirs. As it flowed from one to the other, it intermittently inflated and deflated a cuff round the patient's leg.'

It was, by all accounts, a contraption to behold, and Polak Daniels loved it. Kolff remembers him standing at the end of the patient's bed, his eyes glued as much to the machine as to the man with the failing circulation, never tiring of seeing the flow of water from reservoir to reservoir, the cuff gripping then releasing the patient's leg. Other professors might have been dismissive and told their assistants to spend more time on the proper study of internal medicine and not to fiddle about with a jumble of rubber pipes, but Polak Daniels encouraged Kolff, and their mutual respect sustained Kolff in the troubled times ahead.

The talk throughout Europe was of war. In preparation, doctors were called up into the army, leaving many rural areas with no medical cover. As a last resort health officials took assistants from the universities and sent them to work in the small villages. Kolff was posted to the northern province of Friesland, to a small group of deeply rural villages centred around Sybrandaburen. Although it was only a short distance from Groningen – less than 100 kilometres – in Friesland 'the people are known for their stubbornness, but they're honest and straightforward'.

It is true that Friesland and its people are almost a race apart, and sixty years ago their difference must have been even more noticeable. The region is, coincidentally, also known for its intellectuals and inventors; its people cannot be bluffed and can only be won round with sound logical argument. Kolff was soon to discover this. 'I visited a very old lady who I found lying on a bedstead in one of the villages. I had to give her an intravenous injection. I asked her to stick out her arm. She said that she was so old that she didn't feel her life should be prolonged. My answer was that prolongation of her life was in the hands of the Lord, not mine. Satisfied with that argument, she presented her arm willingly.'

It was winter when he took up his post; it had been very cold, there was snow. This is a landscape of meadows with relatively few trees, and canals along the roadside. In winter these were covered with snow, so it was very hard to see where the road ended and the canal began. The Dutch, for hundreds of years, have had unusual foot-warmers: earthenware pots are placed in wooden boxes and then filled with glowing peat to keep the feet warm while sitting. It is, apparently, particularly useful for women who can drape their robes over the pot to keep themselves warm. To thaw the brakes of his car, Kolff often put the glowing pots under the brakes for the night in the hope that the wheels would run freely in the morning.

Kolff slipped easily into the life of a locum doctor, enjoying the people as much as the classical Dutch landscape. And his patients seem to have enjoyed being treated by him. His friends speak of an easy and reassuring bedside manner, his warm and understanding smile coupled with a medical thoroughness which inspired confidence. He loved the Friesland experience, and the patients. 'I remember one family who had an extremely nice little son of about two-and-a-half years old who decided that he would rather be a girl. Apparently the maid had told him that he could be changed to a girl if he went to the hospital in the neighbouring city of Sneek. So he put his little wooden shoes in the hall, ready to go at any time. I shall never forget him.'

After gathering sufficient experience of 'front-line' medicine, Kolff resumed his work with Polak Daniels in Groningen. The day he was given sole charge of four hospital patients for the first time was the day that defined the remainder of his entire career. Too young and too early in his career to be immune to the death of a patient, Kolff felt a desperate sense of helplessness as he watched a young man of twenty-two, Jan Bruning, die of kidney failure.

Unable to help in any way, Kolff observed the slow and miserable end to this young man's life. His blood pressure soared, his skin itched without mercy as fine crystals of urea – one of the many toxic chemicals which were poisoning his blood and would normally be removed by healthy kidneys – forced their way through his pores. His mother, an elderly country woman dressed in black silk and wearing a white lace cap she had made herself, stood by his bedside. He couldn't see her; the retinas in his eyes were damaged beyond repair. She turned to Kolff and asked 'Is it cancer?' When he told her it wasn't, she thanked God out loud. But Kolff knew this was deadlier than cancer. It was total kidney failure. Bruning was poisoning himself by being unable to rid himself of the toxins his body naturally produced. There was nothing that Kolff could do. He remembers: 'It made an enormous impression on me. And I thought if I could just remove every day as much urea and other products as are normally excreted by the kidneys, then this young man could live.'

It may seem a modest ambition to remove from someone's body the equivalent of a cupped handful of white crystals (which is how urea appears when not in solution), but that apparently simple aim had been attempted before, and with little success. The first efforts were made by three doctors, John Jacob Abel, Leonard Rowntree and B.B. Turner, working in America in 1913. Their experiments involved passing blood (from dogs) through collodion surrounded by a saline solution, and they showed that it was possible to remove substances from the blood through a membrane. The membrane, in this case collodion, was made out of a thick solution of nitro-cellulose in a mixture of alcohol and ether. If the mixture is spread on a surface and the alcohol allowed to evaporate, a thin membrane is left behind. Abel, Rowntree and Turner formed their collodion into tubes. But the major stumbling block for them, and the reason why the first machine to be christened an 'artificial kidney' was never further developed, was the tendency of the blood to clot the instant it entered their apparatus. They had no effective anti-coagulant other than a crude drug, hirudin, which was extracted from leeches, but its side-effects included lung and heart damage as well as allergic reactions. They had successfully tested hirudin as an anti-coagulant in dogs, but it was only when the German researcher Georg Haas tried to use the artificial kidney on wounded German soldiers in the First World War that the drug's adverse reactions in humans were discovered. Abel, Rowntree and Turner might have continued their experiments, according to Abel, had not the leeches been imported from Hungary – where the First World War was becoming more important than the catching of these unprepossessing creatures. Why he didn't buy them locally, in Baltimore where they flourished, he doesn't explain. No matter, they moved on to other areas of research, Abel becoming a pioneer in the crystallising of insulin.

Given the failure of such distinguished medical men before him, what chance then that a young doctor, still under training and fresh from a tiny rural practice, could possibly make any headway towards solving a problem that more experienced minds than his had grappled with? Yet there was hope, possibly because in the intervening years there had been two major advances. The first was the appreciation of the filtering properties of a relatively new substance called cellophane, and the second was the introduction of an anti-coagulant drug called heparin.

Luck also played a not inconsiderable part. Three weeks after Jan Bruning died, a chance meeting took place between Kolff and Professor Robert Brinkman, the first professor of medical biochemistry in Groningen. Brinkman was familiar with cellophane, which he had used successfully as a filter in the commercial purification of fruit juices. Both he and Kolff believed that cellophane was the key to the problem. Unlike the variable quality collodion used by Abel, Rowntree and Turner, which was made by hand, cellophane could be produced in sheets of uniform thickness on a factory scale. But its most important property was that when it was placed between two fluids of different chemical concentrations then molecules of the chemicals that were present in greater quantity on one side moved through the membrane into the solution where they were less concentrated. Things which were too large to pass through the membrane, like protein molecules and blood corpuscles, remained where they were.

Brinkman had seen the potential of cellophane as the basis of an artificial kidney on the strength of those filtering properties alone, and had constructed several of his own prototypes using large, flat sheets of cellophane. One major problem had arisen, though: it was known that only molecules close to the surface of the cellophane were able to pass through, but by presenting as large a surface area as possible to the urea solution (used instead of blood to test the device) Brinkman thought that he could improve the efficiency of the apparatus. A more extreme model used cellophane made into the shape of a nylon stocking, which was draped over a glass rod the size of a leg. The blood, however, could not be persuaded to flow between the glass and the cellophane, and so neither was efficient enough to represent a breakthrough, for reasons Kolff was later to discover.

Kolff took careful note of the fact that if the cellulose membrane acted as a gate, which in effect let the urea and other toxins pass through but did not allow blood to pass, wasn't this the very kind of filter which would have saved Jan Bruning's life? In principle, of course, it was. But this had been recognised by all those who attempted to make an artificial kidney before him, such as Thalimer (a pupil of Dr Abel), who showed in 1938 that cellophane was a suitable basis on which to build an artificial kidney if two major problems could be solved: the first was maintaining a sufficiently large surface area between the blood and the dialysing fluid; the second was to devise a machine that didn't contain so much blood that the patient went into shock. On its own, cellophane was far from being the solution to the problem of removing all the blood from a patient, cleansing it and restoring full health.

Without doubt Kolff would have made no progress had it not been for the invention of cellophane. It was discovered, accidentally, in 1908 by Jacques E. Brandenburger, a Swiss textile engineer who happened to spill his glass of wine across the tablecloth when leaving a restaurant. In a moment of anger came a vision. What the world needed, he decided, was a clear flexible film to protect cloth from soiling and at the same time to make it waterproof. His first attempt involved applying liquid viscose, a cellulose product, directly on to the cloth. This didn't work. The coating simply peeled off again – but in a clear transparent sheet. With this new product in his hands, he forgot all ideas of protecting tablecloths, and pursued new schemes for using this new, transparent film. He called it cellophane, and it was made commercially available for the first time in 1912.

Inspired by the filtering properties of cellophane, Kolff decided to conduct some experiments on himself. He took a sample of his own blood, and added to it 400 mg of urea, thus replicating to some extent the composition of the blood circulating in the body of a patient with kidney failure. He took a tube of cellophane in the form of a 50 cm length of sausage skin and poured the blood/urea mixture into it. He tied the end, then dropped it on to a board immersed in a bath of water. A small motor gave the board a little rocking movement so the blood would move around inside the cellophane tube as the water sloshed around outside it.

After five minutes he removed it and analysed the blood, hardly daring to hope that the urea level would have dropped. To his utter surprise, nearly all the urea had been removed. His mind went into overdrive. He calculated that if he made the cellophane tubing twenty times as long, and could arrange for a patient's blood to pass through it while it was in continuous motion in a bath, then he would have built the first artificial kidney! He conducted a further experiment, this time using a solution of urea in water instead of his own blood, and made careful notes of the results to include them later in his thesis.

It remained a huge leap from a theoretical notion, dreamed up by a young if highly imaginative doctor, to a machine with clinical applications. Many had tried before him and got to precisely this stage, and some of them had even had heparin and cellophane at their disposal. The problem remained a mechanical one, that of contact between blood and dialysing fluid – and not too much blood at that. This was the fundamental problem that Kolff had to solve, and the one which had confounded those before him.

On his own admission Kolff was lucky that the reliable anti-coagulant heparin was also available to him. In 1916, a second-year American medical student in Baltimore, Jay McLean, was working under the direction of William H. Howell, a noted and well respected physiologist whose speciality at the time was blood coagulation, on which subject he was reckoned a world expert. Coincidentally they were working in what in retrospect seems to have been a truly inventive atmosphere at the St John's Hospital, where the medical advances made include the discovery of vitamin D, the identification of three types of polio virus in 1949, the purification of insulin in 1926, and the first ever tissue culture in 1907. It was also the first hospital in the world to use rubber gloves in surgery, back in 1889.

Howell's major discovery up to 1916 had been thrombin, an enzyme active in the final stages of blood coagulation, which he isolated in 1910. Some texts record that he also discovered the drug which had the opposite effect, heparin. But the truth is far from clear. His researcher, Jay McLean, was set the task of finding a way of isolating cephalin, a lipid involved in many of the body's metabolic processes, which had hitherto been extracted only from the brain. In the course of that work, he isolated by accident a compound from the liver which, when tested, had exactly the opposite properties of a coagulant. Thinking it was of little importance to his main line of research, he did not include it in his published work. A couple of years later Howell himself isolated another anti-coagulant from the liver, calling it heparin, and for the rest of his career seemed happy enough to be credited as the discoverer of it, although he never denied McLean's earlier work.

Enter Charles Herbert Best of Toronto, who first isolated insulin. He became the first person to purify heparin into a form in which it was commercially applicable, and you will also see his name recorded as the discoverer of it. Poor old Jay McLean, who may have been the true pioneer, after a lacklustre career partly spent as an ambulance driver in the First World War, waited until Howells had died before he let it be known that the discovery was truly his, a fact that was finally acknowledged in his obituary in the *New York Times*.

So, largely by accident, McLean had provided Kolff with the second ingredient needed to build an artificial kidney – a safe drug to prevent the blood clotting as it flowed through the machine. Nothing, Kolff thought, was going to stop him now. Except possibly the medical establishment. Kolff recalls that 'the head of the assistants became mad, *very* mad when I told him my idea. He thought it was crazy.'

Had not the Second World War intervened, it might not have taken Kolff long to prove how wrong his detractors were, for he was already building contraptions of varying complexity of which he remarks, dryly, 'none of them was clinically applicable'. The events of 10 May 1940, however, put an immediate stop to any further research. The Netherlands was invaded, and the 400,000-strong Dutch army was overwhelmed in a mere five days. It was a walkover – all the more surprising for Holland had always thought itself safe from invasion from the rest of mainland Europe, defended by a marshy expanse of land to the south-west through which tanks were believed to be unable to pass. Hitler's advancing army proved the theory hopelessly wrong, leaving the Netherlands defenceless. As the tanks advanced, German parachutists landed near Rotterdam and The Hague, quickly capturing bridges and airfields to enable transport convoys and planes to bring reinforcements. By first light transport planes were landing, and invading aircraft were using the wide, straight roads as landing strips. By mid-morning the German 18th Army was striking up from the south, capturing that night the rail bridge which had been the Dutch first line of defence. Two days later the German armoured division had made contact with their airborne troops near Rotterdam, and Queen Wilhelmina and her government had retreated to England. On the morning of 14 May the Germans warned that if the Dutch continued to fight, Rotterdam and Utrecht would be destroyed in an air attack. To reinforce the threat, two hours before the deadline expired the Luftwaffe attacked Rotterdam. The entire centre was completely destroyed and thirty thousand civilians died. The country surrendered.

Kolff saw it all with his own eyes. Janke's grandfather Krüseman had died the week before and the funeral was to take place in The Hague, which was regarded as a safe place, given that Holland had remained neutral in the war so far, and was therefore unlikely to be invaded by the Germans. On that basis Pim and Janke thought it safe to leave their one-year-old son Jack with a maid in Groningen and take the train to The Hague on 9 May. It was the last train to reach its destination that night.

They were woken early by the sounds of war: aircraft, bombs, machine-guns. Kolff turned to Janke and said, 'It's war. We might not see Jack for months.' They scrambled up to the flat roof of grandfather's house. Next door were army barracks with gun emplacements, and, oblivious to any danger, they thought it a good place to get a view of what they guessed was the invasion.

They first saw pamphlets rain down from low-flying aircraft, warning all who cared to read them that resistance would be futile. They stood on the roof and looked up and saw one plane trailing a dark column of smoke. Then the pilot parachuted out and the plane came down. 'From where we stood on the flat roof, we couldn't see or hear the soldiers in the barracks, but clearly they saw this plane come down because the next thing we heard was shouts of joy coming up through our roof. Then there was much flak. Bullets ricocheted on the roof, one hit the chimney. That's when we decided to come down.'

The burial of Janke's grandfather, however, had to proceed. But Kolff thought his immediate duty as a doctor was elsewhere. Meanwhile, the funeral was by all accounts the most hurried interment ever. The family had been warned that every moving vehicle was being shot at, so the exercise was conducted at high speed with a dash from home to cemetery and back, Janke trying hard to control her morning sickness – she was pregnant with their second child.

Horrified at the potential for suffering that this raid had brought about, Kolff took himself to the largest hospital in The Hague, where there were large numbers of casualties caused by air strikes on the three military airports nearby in the early hours of 10 May. Kolff had briefly worked in The Hague as a locum during his student days and, knowing the hospital, thought his help might be welcome. He drove at high speed, passing shot-down planes and gliders along the roadside. On arrival at the hospital, his first question was a simple one: do you have a blood bank? When the negative reply came, he said, 'Do you want me to set one up?' This was a revolutionary idea, for the development of blood banks was still in its infancy. The usual practice at the time was for blood to be taken from a donor when needed, and put into an ampoule obtained from the Red Cross in Amsterdam. However, as soon as fighting started on 10 May, roads between The Hague and Amsterdam were blocked, thus giving added importance to Kolff's blood bank.

The world's very first blood bank is reckoned to have been established in a Leningrad hospital in 1932; the first in the USA was in Cook County Hospital, Chicago, in 1937. But the major advance took place in 1940 at the Columbia Presbyterian Hospital, New York, when Dr Charles Drew developed a technique for long-term preservation of blood plasma. He found that by separating the liquid red blood cells from the near solid plasma, and freezing both, they could be reconstituted at a later date. At the same time Karl Landsteiner was discovering the Rh blood group system which he found to be the cause of the adverse reactions that occurred in some transfusions.

Kolff was aware that all these problems might present themselves, and prepared for them. 'If you are going to have a large number of blood transfusions, sooner or later you are going to have a mismatch. That was certainly true of the days when the Rh positive and negative blood groups were not yet known. So even if you had compatible A, B, C and O, you still had the possibility that a Rh negative patient would receive Rh positive blood. A chill and severe haemolysis (red cell breakdown) would be the result, and if you didn't do anything about it the haemoglobin would clog up the renal tubules and the patient might well die of renal failure. To overcome the consequences of mismatch transfusion you can give two litres of 5 per cent glucose intravenously immediately to dilute the large urine output, and you could give 5 per cent sodium bicarbonate to keep the blood alkaline so that the haemoglobin would not precipitate in the urine. Therefore in our blood bank there were always available 2 litres of 5 per cent glucose solution and a bottle of sodium bicarbonate.'

With typical inventiveness, and the hospital's approval, Kolff was given a car and an escort – a soldier who sat on the front seat, clutching a gun to protect them from snipers who now made the streets too dangerous to walk. Carrying a handful of vouchers which the hospital had given him, Kolff drove around the town, at some personal risk, and bought bottles, tubes, needles, citrate and all the paraphernalia required to set up a blood bank. Four days later he was in business with blood, blood plasma and concentrated red blood cells. It was the first ever blood bank on the continent of Europe. 'Maybe it was my lack of familiarity with the English language, but I didn't realise that in English, bank can mean a collection of things. I thought of bank as a money bank. So I arranged my blood bank the way a money bank is run. A doctor could write a cheque and for that cheque he would get a bottle of blood. Then he was in debit and he got a note from the bank, "you are in debit". He could clear his debit if he sent any donor from any blood group to the bank to give a bottle of blood. He could also create a credit by sending donors to the blood bank. This worked very nicely.'

For his work in setting up this blood bank, Kolff was awarded the Landsteiner medal in silver. The experience also gave him a new confidence. 'Handling blood outside the body, as I had to learn to do, helped me later when I had to process blood via the artificial kidney, without doubt.'

The efficiency of his makeshift blood bank, and his grasp of the science of blood transfusion, was soon to be put to the test. On 14 May, only four days after the invasion, Kolff climbed up to the roof of the hospital (the tallest building in the city), to survey the capital of his now-occupied country. 'I saw an enormous mushroom cloud. Yes, a mushroom cloud over Rotterdam! The Germans were attacking it with incendiary bombs. I knew there was no water supply any longer in the city, and so a firestorm soon broke out with such enormous force that a cloud formed, just like the clouds we associate with atomic bombs.' He anticipated that the casualty list would be enormous, so he gathered together his precious blood supplies and drove them the following morning to the remnants of the burnt-out city. The loss of life was less than expected and the demand for blood was not considered urgent. But Kolff had been ready.

He remembers that when things were not going very well in the war and Holland suffered yet another setback, all kinds of rumours made the rounds. It was said that at a small airfield close to The Hague, Germans had landed planes and the airfield commander, still in his pyjamas, had got out of bed and shot at the incoming aircraft. One of them, it was said, carried a German general with a white horse. The story was widely believed.

Satisfied that his blood bank was running efficiently and able to cope, Kolff returned to the comparative peace of the hospital, which maintained its formal atmosphere despite the excitement and the pressures of the outbreak of war. 'There is something special about the atmosphere of a hospital at night. I have always loved it. I made rounds during the night to see if the blood transfusions in the patients that needed them were running satisfactorily. Coming back in one of the dark halls I saw a small group consisting of Professor Michael, who was the head of surgery, and two attractive Red Cross volunteers who were there in case they could give any help. At that time the head nurse, the matron, came in sight, and usually head nurses have great power and people are afraid of them. This was the case with the two Red Cross volunteers. As soon as he saw her approach, Professor Michael, always happier when in close proximity to attractive girls, suggested they stood very close to him for protection. The matron passed, the professor bowed deeply from his waist, and the danger passed by.'

Kolff was to suffer a personal loss at the outbreak of war. Fearful of the German invaders, Professor Polak Daniels, Kolff's mentor and friend, the man who had neither mocked his ideas nor tried to hinder his experiments, committed suicide, as did a number of other Jews who were already aware of the destiny of their race in Hitler's Germany. It was a cruel blow. Kolff had lost his champion, and some years later wrote of him, 'Whereas other members of the staff had shown marked impatience regarding my plans for an artificial kidney, Polak Daniels had allowed me to go ahead without ridiculing the idea. His death left a vacancy.' Kolff had lost a true friend and inspiration.

Polak Daniels's eventual successor was certainly not to Kolff's taste. He was replaced with a loathsome National Socialist with the grandiose German name Kreutz Wendedich von dem Borne – 'a title accorded to the lowest nobility', Kolff remarked with disdain. He hated the National Socialists and their principle that 'those who are not worthy should be killed', and in no circumstances would Kolff work under one. It would have been a betrayal of everything that both he and Polak Daniels believed in. In a rare moment of malice, Kolff says, 'The good Lord helped me and gave the man tuberculosis, and that postponed his coming to Groningen for six months.'

This was just the time Kolff needed to complete his graduation as a specialist in internal medicine. With help from the university administrator, described by Kolff as 'a good Dutchman', his papers were duly signed, thus ensuring that arrest by the Germans was less likely. It was no small coincidence that Kolff's leaving date was given as the day before the despised Kreutz Wendedich von dem Borne took up his post.

Kolff remembers with some delight that a year later a reunion of former assistants at Groningen university was held. When he and his young assistant Bob van Noordwijk were entering the city the police drew them to the side of the road. A funeral procession approached, bound for the cemetery. Bob remembers that on the coffin stood a National Socialist cap, wobbling: 'Kolff broke into a laugh and said, "I left Groningen when *he* arrived here, now he is going out when *I* am coming in".' Kolff later added, 'I have never stood with more satisfaction along a road, seeing a funeral procession, as when his coffin passed by.'

4

A NEW MISSION –
TO MAKE PEOPLE SICK!

Kolff first came to the small city of Kampen, in the north-east of Holland, in August 1940. Of the seven candidates interviewed for the vacancy for a specialist in internal medicine at the city's hospital, he was the youngest, and the only one with the audacity to make demands before even being offered the post. He first insisted that there should be improvements to the X-ray machine, and certainly that it should be replaced by one more sophisticated than that housed in the nearby town of Zwolle. He also announced that before he would consider the job he required an electrocardiograph, and most important of all he needed a proper clinical laboratory, complete with assistants, if he were to do his work properly. It was an aggressive stance for the youngest of the candidates, but his interview technique clearly worked and he was appointed from 1 July 1941 with 'all demands met'.

Kampen Hospital was a modest setting for a major medical breakthrough. The city itself had only 23,000 residents when Kolff came to work there alongside the hospital's only surgeon. It remains a small city with a self-sufficient feel, its ancient heart and cobbled streets protected by medieval walls, gates and towers. It has an imposing town hall, a medieval magistrates' court, a clock tower complete with carillon of forty-seven bells, and a nineteenth-century waterfront where the old sailboats of the 'brown fleet' still lean graciously against the quayside. Its tobacco museum, which gives a hint as to the basis of its former prosperity, boasts the largest cigar in the world. The town's heyday was in the fourteenth and fifteenth centuries, when it was one of the most powerful and wealthy towns in the whole of the Netherlands due to its position at the mouth of the River Ijssel, a major finger of the vast Rhine delta. It was a Hanseatic town, a member of a group of influential trading ports which stretched across a large part of northern Europe from Holland through the Baltic states and eventually to Latvia and Estonia. Through these ports came wine, beer and honey, timber, wax and animal skins to satisfy the needs of the growing European population. Citrus fruits came by ship from Spain and Portugal, clothes from Italy. Kampen could count itself among the major ports, such as Hamburg, Lubeck, Gdansk, Riga and Brugge. In trading terms it is a shadow of its former self, but its pride remains tangible to this day.

By the time Kolff arrived to take up his post in July 1941, with his wife and two children (the second, Adrie, having been born in November of the previous year), Kampen remained a place apart from the oppressive and restrictive atmosphere of that occupied country. 'There was a part of the city where cows were still living in stables inside people's houses in the winter when the meadows were flooded. They were scrupulously clean. The tails of the cows were tied to a rope which passed over a pulley in the roof; to the other end of the rope was attached a weight. As the cows got up and down, their tails never dropped into the manure. Spotless. They even cooked in the same room as the cows, and slept above them. Hay was kept in the top floor of the houses and I saw it being thrown down to the animals in the streets.' It was once said of Kampen that its hapless people have a tendency towards stupidity, for they never acquired the wit or speed of mind to get out of the way of the revolving sails of the windmills, and the repeated blows to their heads took its toll on their intelligence.

Strict religious views held sway when Kolff first arrived. He remembers it as a community of reformed Protestants: 'brave and willing people who would do anything to help you if you needed it, because God expected it of them. But don't try to borrow a bicycle pump on a Sunday because they'd have nothing to do with you. I remember an old farmer coming in for an X-ray and being asked to remove all his clothes. This he did, except for his hat. He understood modesty.'

Home for the Kolffs was a small, semi-detached house in Jan van Arkel Straat in a neat and tidy housing estate, no more than ten minutes' walk from the hospital. This was their family home for nearly nine years, and life here was no luxurious experience. 'Food was scarce, fuel even more difficult to come by. Often in those bleak wartime winters we would wake to find the water in the kettle frozen solid, or ice crystals shimmering on the damp walls.' As well as a home, the house had to serve as a refuge – a hiding-place where Kolff could escape the occupying Germans if necessary. At the top of a spiral staircase, which led to the loft where apples and carrots were stored to feed them through the winter, there was a cavity beneath the eaves, no more than a tiny triangular space in a gap between the slope of the roof and the outside walls. 'That is where I would hide if the Germans ever came for me. I could run up the two flights of stairs, crawl into that hiding-place, and close the shutter behind me before Janke had answered the door. Every time we heard the sound of boots in the street at night we were afraid. When a car stopped, you knew it was likely that you or one of your neighbours was going to be arrested. They'd take hostages. Sometimes they'd shoot them and leave the bodies on the street corners. They shot the surgeon in a nearby town, you know.'

Indeed, Kolff's own life could have depended on a fine calculation which was well rehearsed. 'It would take me one minute and thirty seconds precisely to get into that hiding-place, if I had to. None of this means I wasn't afraid', Kolff insists. 'I often went home and looked at Janke and the children and imprinted them on my mind so I'd have something to remember if I were ever in prison. We both said that if either of us were taken prisoner, even if they tortured us we'd never give away anything we knew. We agreed that.'

Fifty years later, Jack Kolff was to write of his early memories in wartime Kampen. 'Parents will shield their children from the realities of war and protect them from fear. We children thought it normal to stand in line at the soup kitchens and trade coupons for soup ladled into the family's bucket. We considered it normal to see helmeted troops in the streets, to draw the shades at night, to watch dog-fights in the air, to play in a bomb shelter with the neighbourhood children, and to listen to the drone of bombers overhead. No sooner was the last out of earshot, than another squadron would approach to deliver revenge on the nation that took so many lives.'

Battle was being waged on many fronts in Kampen. Apart from the military resistance against the Germans orchestrated by the Allies, a more subtle war was also being played out by heroic individuals who risked their lives to publish underground newspapers, or give aid to Jews or students who refused to sign a declaration of allegiance to the Germans. Resistance groups were active throughout the Netherlands led by the Dutch government in exile, which operated from London and organised drops of weapons to be used against the Germans.

Kolff had potent weapons other than guns at his disposal though, and paradoxically found himself having to reverse his medical principles. Instead of making people well, he had to make them appear ill, or at least the victims of medical circumstances outside their control. For example, when food became scarce (much of the produce from Holland's fertile farmland was exported to Germany, leaving the Dutch to starve) a system of ration cards was established. The problem was obtaining a ration card for someone who was in hiding, who might be a Jew or a suspected resistance worker who dared not show their face. Some were former soldiers in the defeated Dutch army who were tricked by the Germans when they were offered an amnesty; it was, in fact, a deception to gather former soldiers so they could be deported to the work camps. Those who didn't fall for this trick went swiftly into hiding, but all needed food, and to get food required a ration card.

The solution, devised by the resistance workers, was to form a series of 'hit squads' who would raid the rationing offices and steal ration cards at gunpoint. Kolff remembers that at one such office, just across the water from Kampen, the Dutch manager wanted nothing more than to help his fellow countrymen and to release as many ration cards as they wanted, but if he made it appear too easy he would be shot by the Germans. He went to see Kolff. 'He said he wanted to be anaesthetised so that when the Germans came to question him he could honestly say the raiders had put him to sleep and he didn't remember a thing.' Kolff duly provided him with a mask and a bottle of ether. 'He was never arrested.'

Not all the resistance's ideas were practicable ones, though. 'They decided that the resistance people should all have identification cards so that they could identify themselves to each other, and eventually to the Allies when they came.' It was a well-intentioned if dangerous idea. 'In Apeldoorn, they caught one person, saw his identity card, and through him found the head of the resistance whom they then shot and dropped on a street corner with a few others to teach the underground a lesson. I refused to have anything to do with identity cards. I didn't want my name on any list. Nothing was in writing and the only person you knew in the resistance was the one above you. That way, if you were captured, there was very little information you could be forced to give away, even if they tortured you. It was best to know very little.' However, Kolff remained close to the resistance, obtaining scarce petrol ration cards to pass to other doctors. He remembers the telephone network which linked resistance workers. The code worked like this: on calling the operator at the Kampen exchange, he would ask the simple question, 'How is your daughter?' If the reply came that she was 'not well, doctor', Kolff knew it was unsafe for him to speak because the Germans were listening in. If the reply came that she was in the finest health, it was safe for him to pass information to the operator, who would relay it. 'I met that telephone operator only after the liberation', remembers Kolff. 'It was strange to see him for the first time because he wasn't at all how I imagined him. He was elderly, had no teeth, but a wonderful smile.'

The most coveted document became the 'Ausweiss': a declaration that you were unfit for work on medical grounds and therefore of no use to the Germans. It was the only guarantee against deportation. Kolff got many requests. 'I remember a man called Domingo, an engineer working on land reclamation, and being a scientist he had a flame photometer, a very new piece of equipment at the time. I knew that if I had access to that I could use it to determine potassium levels in the blood of my patients, which was of great importance in determining their kidney function. This was quite new technology. Not even the universities had these machines. Anyway, he came to me because he had been told by the Germans that he was to join a gang of people digging fox-holes.' These so-called fox-holes were trenches for Germans to crawl into if there were an invasion, though sometimes the digging of them was only an excuse to gather together fit men who found that, once they had dug one fox-hole, there was a one-way lorry waiting to take them to Germany where they would have to dig more. The Germans were also nervous that too many fit men might remain in Holland, every able-bodied man being a potential freedom fighter, and digging fox-holes kept them not only occupied but under close observation.

Kolff recalls, 'I decided to help him because by allowing me use of his flame photometer he could help my patients. I gave him picric acid. It makes you yellow. The man looked as though he had jaundice. If you're a specialist then the yellow is actually a different shade from the colour you go when you've got liver failure, but any doctor who took a quick look at this man would say he had jaundice, no doubt about it. He looked so ill after I had "treated" him that he had no problem getting his Ausweiss.'

Kolff also remembers the day a man who went by the name 'Uncle Joe' appeared at his hospital. He was suffering from a not uncommon condition at the time – fear. He was the head of the local resistance, and word had reached him through the underground that he was about to be arrested. He needed to be ill, he decided, and pleaded with Kolff that he would be safe from arrest if he were safely tucked up in a hospital bed. It called for Kolff's fine judgement. There was no way of verifying that he was indeed a resistance worker, since Kolff's stated principle had been 'only to know the one above you'. It could have been a double-cross to expose Kolff. In the end, after hearing the man's pleas, Kolff decided he was trustworthy. 'I always had to be extremely careful. We had one nurse in the hospital who was certainly a National Socialist and there was always the threat that she would talk about what she'd seen, although to her credit she never did. So, with my head nurse, who I knew would *never* betray us, I carefully took Uncle Joe, put him into bed and took a litre of his blood. Then I gave him a stomach tube and by putting a funnel on the end of it, I poured the blood back into him. I then told him he had a bleeding ulcer and stood over him while he learned the symptoms so he could describe them to anyone who asked. Then I asked for laboratory tests to be done in the usual way. Of course, they found blood in his stool sample, and his haemoglobin levels were low because of the amount of blood I had taken from him. There was only one clinical conclusion – he had a bleeding ulcer. Uncle Joe was never arrested. He stayed in the hospital bed until the threat was past.'

It became nothing unusual for Kolff to make people convincingly ill. He admitted a Pole, a conscript in the German army, and the surgeon removed his appendix although there was no need to. When this didn't convince the Germans that the Pole was unfit to serve in the army, Kolff gave him the symptoms of tuberculosis, even administering a drug into his bronchial tubes to ensure that the required shadows would appear on the upper right lobes of the Pole's lung in an X-ray. Tuberculosis was the disease the Germans feared more than anything else, so another 'patient' was off the hook.

The nearest Kolff came to refusing to help the fight

against the Germans happened after a farmer named Post arrived at the hospital and announced, 'Dr Kolff, we are in trouble. I know of a small street where a lady there is hiding two Jewish women, and one of them is going to die. We need your help.' This plea came as no surprise to Kolff and Janke, for they had already given help in the past by providing blankets and sheets, carefully ensuring that any of the hospital's laundry marks were removed. He had analysed a sputum sample from the sick woman, who was spitting blood in large quantities, and knew she was riddled with tuberculosis. But Post had not come to plead for a cure. He simply asked, 'What are we going to do with the body when she's dead?' To arrive in the street with his wagon to remove the body would have revealed to the Germans the guilt of the woman who had given refuge to the Jews. A curfew prevented the body being moved under the cover of darkness. Kampen is a town of narrow streets and alleys with front doors opening directly on to those streets, and it was impossible to keep *anything* secret, certainly not the removal of a body. 'There is only one way I know of to remove that body', said Post. Kolff feared what was coming next.

Post explained that it was not unusual for people to sell items of furniture during the war in order to buy food or fuel. Post had agreed with the householder that he would buy a cabinet from her, then arrive in broad daylight with his wagon, load it up, and take it away. There would be nothing suspicious about that. No one would guess there was a body in it. 'Only one problem,' Post explained. 'The body will be too big. Will you come and cut it up for us? I am a farmer. If it were a sheep or a pig I would have no problem. But I've never cut up a human body.'

Kolff knew how serious this situation was. The head of the Kampen police, a National Socialist, was a man of little compassion. He would certainly arrest the old lady who had provided shelter to the Jews and deport her without compunction to Germany to be treated as if she were a Jew herself. Kolff was aware that a Jewish girl of only twelve had recently been discovered in hiding just across the river, and the father and four sons who had sheltered her were dispatched to work camps. No word had been heard of them since, and they were presumed dead.

'I didn't look forward to cutting up the body, but I felt it was my duty to help them. I enquired if there was a flush toilet, which was essential so I could get rid of the blood. There was. Post went away saying he would call me when the woman had died. I waited and waited, but thankfully no message ever came. I was dreading having to do it. Later, after the liberation, when the war was over, I was on my bicycle when I heard a woman calling my name. I got off and a lady came across and shook my hand and introduced herself as the lady who had harboured the two Jews. She introduced me, and I shook hands with the woman I had promised to cut up. I assume she never heard about our arrangement. I hope not.'

Kolff never missed an opportunity to rob the Germans of a potential prisoner. He played a delicate psychological game with the occupiers, trying to persuade them that 'the sick are no use to you, let me take them'. And in return for his dedication, those around offered theirs: nurses made him milky drinks, or put him into a hospital bed for a few short hours to get valuable rest. He remembers, 'Sometimes I was so tired, I just went home and cried'.

After making a life as best he and Janke could for their two children, assembling his medical team came next on his agenda. These were to be the people who could fill the gaps in the hospital's structure and transform it from a centre for the treatment of the sick into a place that could also embrace the research and development work Kolff needed in order to construct his artificial kidney. Over the following months he recruited many people who were to become good friends and close allies, and he was to create the only hospital laboratory in the whole of the Netherlands where determinations could be carried out at any time of the day or night. Mieneke van der Leij, an attractive and highly intelligent woman whom Kolff knew from Groningen, where she had trained in laboratory work, was the first chemical technician to join his team. It had been yet another of Kolff's stipulations that she be allowed to work alongside him at Kampen Hospital. The second to join in January 1943 was Jacob (Bob) van Noordwijk, who was to become a trusted ally and close friend throughout a long and bitter war.

Young Bob had been a student at Groningen in 1938, studying medicine, and would have taken his bachelor's exams in 1941 had he not been arrested by the Gestapo in March of that year for activities unsympathetic to the Germans. He had, in fact, been active in an underground student newspaper. 'I should have been more careful and burned my papers, but I didn't. We were still too innocent at that time.' He was sentenced to eighteen months' imprisonment, and on his release he found his name on a list of students who were no longer allowed to study because of their anti-German activities. Strangely enough, this did not prevent him taking examinations, and so he continued his studies at home, graduating in 1943.

Unable to finish his medical studies, he had to look for work, and went for advice to one of the men he could trust, the biochemist Professor Brinkman. He was unaware of the link between Brinkman and Kolff. Brinkman suggested Kolff might need help at Kampen with his work on the artificial kidney. The alternative was to work in Nijmegen as an assistant to the pathologist, where Bob's duties would be to assist in autopsies. This was the more attractive option because to pass his next medical examinations he would have had to attend 200 autopsies, and by working alongside the pathologist this would be easily achieved. Bob van Noordwijk wrote: 'I visited both Kolff in Kampen and the pathologist in Nijmegen, and on the way back I decided to accept the latter. I had caused a lot of trouble to my parents by my imprisonment and I felt a moral duty to finish my studies after the war as rapidly as possible. I wrote to Kolff, thanking him for the way he had received me in Kampen, but I also told him that I had decided to go to Nijmegen. That evening I regretted that letter deeply. Was it really so important to add another physician to the enormous number there already? But if I went to Kampen I might perhaps assist in the development of a completely new possibility in medicine. The house where I had a room had no telephone, but at the corner of the street there was a shop that did have one. As soon as it opened I went there and phoned Kolff. I told him I had written him a letter with my decision to prefer Nijmegen, but I asked if I could go back on that. "Yes, provided you do it damn quickly", was his reaction. "Can I start work with you on Monday?" I asked. "Yes", was his answer.' The inventive Kolff and the young, contemplative van Noordwijk were to prove a potent combination.

Kolff remembers Nannie van de Leeuw as being useful in his laboratory because of her ability to make precise water-colour paintings of blood cells as seen under the microscope. She first heard of Kolff's work from a newspaper article and thought it sounded interesting. 'I was looking for a job because the Germans had closed my university and I decided to go for an interview. There were no trains, so I cycled. When I got to Kampen I was deeply shocked by Kolff's manner. His first question was, "Are you a Nazi?" "No!" I insisted. I was disgusted by the question. It was a terrible thing to ask. I think he must have seen the look on my face because he apologised and explained he had to be careful because he worked with the underground.' Indeed, Kolff was already enmeshed in a secret web whose aim was to destabilise the Germans, giving help to loyal Dutchmen and women brave enough to grasp an opportunity to score any victory over the invaders. Yet out of the pressures of wartime came close friendships. Nannie van de Leeuw remembers, 'He was lovely to work with, despite the pressures on him. He was very polite when asking you to do things. It was always, "Would you have time to . . .?" We all worked hard, but he was kind to us. He would even lend his car to the girls so they could go and see their fiancées.'

Kampen was well outside the main theatre of war in western Europe and was never heavily bombed, although the great set-piece battles of 1944 around Nijmegen and Arnhem were to take place less than fifty miles away. Kolff remembers the destruction of the Ruhr dams by the British 'Dambusters', not from news reports but rather from the mass of debris that suddenly appeared, floating downstream on the Ijssel river as it passed through Kampen.

Although it was a comparatively safe city in which to work, nevertheless a multitude of small but significant battles were taking place in which Kolff was involved. One of the more audacious was the plot to assassinate the Nazi head of police in Kampen. The plan involved placing an innocent-looking artist, complete with easel, by the attractive old town gate which leads off the road running by the Ijssel river. The distinguished city gate was a favourite subject for painters, and one more artist would not look out of place. It was well known to the Dutch resistance that the head of police swept through these gates daily in his official car and always at the same time. On the chosen day, however, the artist would be no innocent painter but an assassin. Kolff's part in the plot was to lend his car to a getaway driver who would whisk the killer swiftly into the countryside, where he could disappear. However, the plan was confounded on the day the shooting was to take place, when the Nazi's car happened to be accompanied by an outrider; the assassin decided that even if he managed to shoot the chief of police, his chances of escape would be minimal. He decided not to fire but instead took up his easel and walked away. Still afraid that the plot might be discovered, he begged Kolff to drive him out of town as if the assassination had taken place. At no small risk to himself, Kolff obliged.

The challenges presented to Kolff by the war would have tested the strengths and talents of any doctor, let alone one whose already crowded mind repeatedly returned to his notion of building the world's first artificial kidney machine. It is difficult to imagine worse conditions in which to attempt a medical breakthrough.

5

POTS, PANS AND A SPLASHING MACHINE

Kolff's idea of building an artificial kidney that would replicate the myriad functions of the natural kidney must have seemed ridiculous at the time. His early apparatus, brought from Groningen, appeared to be no more than a hopeless contraption of sausage skins and tubes built on a ramshackle metal framework. Indeed, even one of his close and faithful workers, on first seeing it, took a deep breath and exclaimed 'Oh, my God!', hardly able to believe that it was Kolff's intention to connect this paraphernalia to a human being with the intention of drawing their blood through it.

But if his close colleagues remained loyal, some in the hospital administration harboured serious doubts about the game Kolff was playing. 'Messing around' was how some of them viewed his artificial kidney development, clearly believing the forty patients under his care would be better served if a portion of his mind was not dwelling on the belief that a clanking machine of his own invention could replicate the hugely complex workings of the human kidney. The hospital surgeon, Kehrer, scornfully remarked that Kolff was 'playing with kidneys', although he was never deliberately obstructive.

To arouse the suspicions of the doubters even further, he had arrived from Groningen with what amounted to a lifetime's supply of American sausage skins, which was hardly the behaviour of a rational doctor. Kolff remembers, with a smile of satisfaction, 'At the beginning of the war, I paid for a large quantity of sausage skins. When they asked why I needed so much, I joked that we had a famine in Holland. It was quite a lot of sausage skin, I have to admit. Even so, I ran out and had to buy German skins, made in Wiesbaden, but it wasn't as good as the American.'

On his own admission, he 'wakes at four in the morning with an idea, and that's it! Problem solved. I would get up and sit at my desk in the bitter cold, because there was no heating, and I had to write down my idea for fear it would be gone by breakfast.' One morning in 1942, he woke early, before dawn, got dressed and then took to the streets – the solution to the problem which had prevented any further progress had finally come to him. His dilemma had been simple: he knew from the experiment carried out on a sample of his own blood in his Groningen laboratory that in order for urea to pass from the blood through the cellophane and into the dialysing fluid (which was the principal effect he was seeking in his artificial kidney), both the blood and the fluid had to be in continuous motion. Also, the transfer must take place over as large a surface area as possible, and the quantity of blood involved must be the absolute minimum. It was the latter two requirements that had partially defeated those before him, notably the Americans Abel, Rowntree and Turner in 1912, and also Professor Brinkman.

Although Kampen was under strict curfew at night, and anyone walking the streets before dawn was likely to be arrested and closely interrogated, Kolff knew he was safe taking an early morning walk. Although he steadfastly refused to aid the Germans in any way, he remarked, 'Although I had nothing to do with them, I had to work with the German doctors because they referred

German soldiers to our hospital. Also I had to be on the good side of the German soldiers to protect myself from the Burgermeister, who was a National Socialist and a nasty man.' As usual, Kolff was treading a careful path through the politics and conflicts of life in wartime Holland. Even so, he must have hoped his dawn wanderings would go unnoticed or ignored by the patrolling German soldiers.

That morning he had an appointment with Hendrik Berk, the owner of a local enamel works, and his mechanic, Mr E.C. van Dijk. The Kampen Enamel Works produced pots and pans by traditional methods. Kolff and Berk had already had a brief discussion at Berk's home about the possibility of building an artificial kidney, but Berk thought van Dijk might have ideas to offer, and so the dawn meeting was arranged. The factory, of course, was forbidden to carry out work for anyone other than the Germans without express permission, and was operating under the watchful eye of a German officer. But knowing that he never reported for duty before eight in the morning, Kolff was confident that a visit before breakfast would be safe from Nazi observation, providing Kolff was clear of the factory by eight.

Kolff outlined an idea that had previously been tried by Brinkman in Groningen. In order to spread the blood over as large an area as possible, and therefore provide the maximum contact with the dialysing fluid, the cellophane tube would be wound round a stainless steel drum which would hang vertically in a bath filled with a saline solution. In order to move the blood through the tube, alongside this drum would be a smaller roller, covered with soft rubber, which would press gently against the cellophane tubing. As the drum and roller rotated, so the blood would be forced through the tubing. It seemed at the time that it might be the answer to all the problems, and certainly it appeared to achieve contact between the blood and the bath fluids over the maximum possible surface area, so that as the blood flowed through, the urea and other toxins would pass through the cellophane membrane into the dialysing fluid, and out of the blood, exactly as Kolff had shown in that simple experiment on his own blood. As to the construction of the machine, Kolff considered it 'not an engineering feat of any difficulty'.

But such a design had been tried and it had never worked. Kolff and Berk were looking for a new idea, and solutions to some difficult problems. First, stainless steel was difficult to obtain, and finding roller bearings that would work in a corrosive saline solution was a problem, too. 'We sat round a table and began to draw', Kolff remembers. 'I already had an idea of what I wanted, but in order for the engineers to feel involved, I let the idea come out of our discussion. The solution we came up with, which Berk thought was his idea, was simply to mount the rotating drum horizontally. He had some thoughts of patenting the design, but when I explained that something similar was already on my mind, he withdrew without question. He was a gentleman.'

To the engineering minds of Berk and van Dijk, the solution was instantly clear. Instead of mounting the revolving drum vertically, it should instead rotate horizontally, like a waterwheel, with only the lower part immersed in the fluid bath, with the result that the bearings would stand clear of the fluid. Also, by suggesting a horizontal rather than a vertical rotation of the drum, they had made a simple but fundamental change to Kolff's original idea – they had solved the problem of achieving a flow of blood through the cellophane tubing without any mechanical help.

Imagine the spiral of cellophane tubing, the sausage skin, as a coiled hose-pipe. Pour, say, half a cupful of water into the hose-pipe and it will immediately fall to the bottom of the first loop, and stay there. Slowly rotate the coiled pipe and watch what happens to that water. As anyone who has tried to empty a coiled garden hose will know, the water will make its own way along the tube until it emerges at the other end. It needs no pump; no pressure of any kind need be applied. As long as the coil rotates, the liquid will eventually emerge at the far end.

What more could Kolff have asked for? In removing completely the need to force the blood through the machine, he had largely eliminated another potential problem – haemolysis, or mechanical damage to the red blood cells, which was largely caused by the destructive action of the pump. This new approach required no pump and almost entirely eliminated the problem at a stroke. All other criteria had been fulfilled. Berk said he would build the machine, and Kolff anxiously awaited its arrival in Kampen Hospital, where it would be installed in his office. It was delivered, presumably through some secret subterfuge, at which Kolff was now becoming accomplished.

The only remaining problem was paying for it. It is doubtful that any of the hospital's budget would have been made available for an unproved device when wartime demands were stretching resources to the limits. By this stage of the war Kampen was without coffee, tea, chocolate and sugar, although some doctors could rely on an illicit supply of milk from grateful farmer patients. The diet consisted largely of cabbage and potatoes, and the bread ration was half a loaf per person per week. This was no time for a hospital to be spending speculative money on Kolff's fanciful machines. Kolff remembers, 'My salary at the time was 10,000 guilders, and that was quite a lot of money in those days. I decided that financial problems would not get in the way of building this machine, even if I had to pay for it myself. I told Berk that the bill should be sent to me.'

But no invoice was ever to arrive. The Kampen Enamel Factory was under German occupation and it was entirely forbidden for Berk to carry out work for anyone other than the Germans. An invoice to Kolff would have given the game away. There remains to this day an outstanding debt on the world's first ever artificial kidney.

But the artificial kidney owes a debt, of a kind, to Janke Kolff too, for after the death of her grandfather Krüseman, she again inherited a substantial sum. Kolff himself has said that he could not have built the kidney machine without the help of a rich wife.

One mechanical problem remained, but this was eventually solved by Kolff's typical ability for lateral thought. What neither he nor Berk had fathomed was how the blood, entering through a fixed tube, could be directed into the rotating tube of sausage skin without leaking. The drum around which the tubing was wrapped rotated, and so, if the blood could pass into the central shaft, the cellophane tubing might then easily be attached to that. But the coupling of a rotating shaft with a blood-tight stationary one presented them with a problem. After a little thought, and possibly yet another dawn inspiration, Kolff reasoned that what he was asking of this coupling was that it should perform the same function as the water pump coupling which he'd seen used in the cooling system of a Ford motor car. He went to the local Ford dealer to examine the spare part, and with a little drilling and slight modification his problem was solved. He remarked, 'The packing around a rotating joint good enough for a Ford automobile would certainly be good enough for an artificial kidney.' His kidney machine, of course, was growing increasingly bizarre – it now consisted of sausage skin, an enamel bath from the local saucepan manufacturer and a Ford water pump. The framework was of aluminium salvaged from a shot-down German bomber. Despite the machine's obvious ingenuity, Berk, reportedly, 'didn't see the potential of it'.

It was finally delivered to Kampen Hospital in October 1942. Set against the background of an ever bloodier war in Europe, it might have seemed something of an irrelevance. A couple of months earlier the gassing of Jews at Auschwitz had commenced (although this was not known in the Netherlands at the time), and the Germans had advanced on Stalingrad. These were days for survival, not for experiment and innovation. But as the war grew ever more oppressive, Kolff grew more determined. I once asked him if the wartime atmosphere had restricted him in any way. He replied, 'No. When I decide to do something, nothing stops me.'

He now had his kidney machine, as yet untested. In 1944 his paper entitled 'The Artificial Kidney: a Dialyser with a Great Area', published in Scandinavian, Dutch and French medical journals to prevent the Germans from claiming the invention as their own, described the machine to the world for the first time. In a later publication, in 1946, 'New Ways of Treating Uraemia', he gave a detailed account of further developments, although the machinery he describes here does not differ greatly from the first.

A big cylinder turns with its undermost segment through a tank with rinsing-liquid. Round this cylinder a long cellophane tube has been spirally wound. The tube contains only a small quantity of blood. This blood sinks by gravity always to the lowest point of the spiral line.

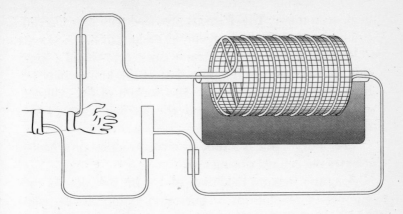

When the cylinder rotates, the blood runs through the spiral line from left to right, always sinking to the lowest point. It enters and leaves the cylinder through the hollow axles, in each of which is fixed a rotating coupling. By connecting the take-up and exhaust tubes with each other, a closed circuit is formed in which the blood circulates rapidly; air bubbles are dragged along.

Then, to prove how essentially simple this machine was and how he still believed he had been correct in describing it as no major feat of engineering, he gave construction details. He made the building of an artificial kidney sound simple enough for a home handyman to accomplish it:

The cylinder . . . is made of varnished lathing. The laths have been screwed on two wooden wheels and project 5 cms. over the wheel at the end of the cylinder. The cylinder turns with its lower segment through a tank with rinsing-liquid, and has two short hollow axles, through which the blood is brought in and led out.

The iron frame: the hollow axles of the cylinder turn in two plain open bearings, which are fitted on a rectangular angle-iron frame. This frame is provided with legs and can be lifted with the cylinder from the underframe.

Resting on ratchets, the frame can rotate round a long side, so that the whole upper part of the kidney may be turned up with the cylinder. The bottom of the cylinder can be well seen then, and the bath can be easily refreshed or cleaned.

The under-frame is a tube-iron construction on wheels; it bears the enamel rinsing tank.

A motor (sewing machine) of 1/4 hp will do. As the number of revolutions of our motors amounts to from 1500 to 3000, this must be converted to 35–50 revolutions per minute with a reduction transmission.

In the rinsing-tank is a heating element. We used the bottom of electrical kettles.

Its essential simplicity is testament to Kolff's abiding belief that there need be nothing too advanced or expensive about an artificial kidney. The next step, though, was to prove that it worked and that it was more than a fanciful collection of tubes, metal and woodwork – which is what it undoubtedly appeared to be at first glance. To achieve a proper clinical trial over the autumn and winter of 1942 and into the early months of 1943, he turned to the next crucial phase of the construction, which was putting the finishing touches to the team of people who would prove to the world that it worked.

He had already turned his modest laboratory into a centre of excellence. He had carefully trained Mieneke van der Leij in the basic but often painstaking tests which she would have to conduct on the patient's blood during the course of any dialysis. Some tests were lengthy, particularly the determination of potassium levels, and most were 'test tube' work – automated analysis was still some decades away. This was more work than one loyal assistant could manage.

Willy Eskes joined the team to share the laboratory's ever increasing workload, and became one more vital assistant in the development of the artificial kidney. She remembers, 'On Saturdays, he'd say "take my car" (only doctors were allowed petrol) or he'd push aside a bottle of urine I was working on and he'd say, "I know what's wrong with him. Let's go skating." He was the sort of man who saw problems from your point of view and put himself in your position.' In fact, the hospital's tight budget did not run to paying for two assistants for Kolff, and Willy Eskes's salary came directly out of Kolff's pocket for a time. 'It was always an adventure to assist him,' she remembers. ' I admired his ideas, I wanted to be part of them, part of his big adventure.'

Versatility was undoubtedly a requirement for working alongside Kolff. Bob van Noordwijk was lucky enough to possess a simple, portable typewriter: 'It served us admirably in writing the first papers on the artificial kidney. It was a great advantage to Kolff that he did not have to do the typing himself, because the person typing the text is more reticent in making changes than the person who leaves the typing to someone else, because not a single word could be crossed out or inserted or moved to another place in the sentence without leaving a trace (I had no correction fluid at my disposal). Typing without errors was a skill that was held in very high esteem at that time – any change in the text meant that the page had to be typed again before a neat final version was reached. Something one never heard was "Just make a copy, will you?" Simple photocopying machines did not exist. Kolff had bought a machine himself and had it installed in the darkroom of the X-ray room of the hospital. It used light-sensitive paper that had to be exposed, developed, fixed, washed and dried to provide a negative. Washing lines along the wall of the darkroom were used to dry the sheets. Persons entering the darkroom when we were busy were often shocked at so many pieces of paper. This was because the copies usually had solemn black borders and looked like death announcements, which were common on the front pages of the newspapers when someone had been killed, often a member of the resistance.'

Although Kolff was now in possession of his first machine, and had the people to help him run it, many problems remained. The purpose of dialysis was not only to remove excess urea from the bloodstream. It was common for patients in kidney failure to suffer a complete imbalance of electrolytes in the blood stream. These electrolytes, such as sodium, potassium, chloride and bicarbonate, are required to be in a precise balance in a healthily functioning body. This fine balancing act was normally the job of the kidney, and it would have to be the job of Kolff's artificial kidney too. Consequently much of his early work centred on using the right mixtures in the dialysing bath. He decided that for his first dialysis, according to his thesis, he would use a solution consisting of 6.5 g of sodium chloride, 2.5 g of sodium bicarbonate, and 0.18 g of potassium chloride per litre of water. These carefully weighed salts were placed in the bottom of the enamel bath built by Berk, and mixed with 70 litres of tepid tap water. As Kolff explained to me, 'You hope to achieve a balance between the salts of the dialysing fluid and the salts in the blood. For example, if the sodium level in the patient's bloodstream is too low, then sodium will pass through the cellophane from the fluid into the blood in the opposite direction to the poisons you are trying to get rid of. If the blood concentration of sodium is too high, the reverse will happen. It all works towards an equilibrium.' He broke off for a laugh, then announced, 'You don't have to be very clever to dialyse, fortunately.'

But all this remained theoretical until the machine could be connected to a patient, and that this could be achieved was far from certain. Kolff's intention was that the blood could be collected by inserting a glass tube into an artery, and returned to a vein by a similar tube. At this stage it was not his ambition to have the patient's blood in continuous flow through the machine. Rather, a quantity of blood would be removed, dialysed and returned to the body. Then further blood would be taken, and so on. It was never envisaged that a kidney machine would be able to provide long-term life support. Kolff's idea was that the machine would provide the patient's own kidneys with some 'relief' and allow them to recover their natural function. The notion that chronic kidney patients might use these machines for years and live normal lives was not yet part of anyone's thinking.

The removal of arterial blood was nothing new, but doubt arose over what would happen to the blood once it had been through the glass and rubber tubing. Kolff was well aware that by giving heparin he could ensure the passage of the blood through the machine without the risk of clotting. But once the dialysis was over, and the blood needed to clot again to prevent bleeding, what would happen then? Wouldn't it leave the patient vulnerable to haemorrhage at the point where the blood left and re-entered the body? Also, the closing of the wounds would be made that much more difficult. Coupled with the possibility of internal bleeding in an already sick patient, the use of heparin without an antidote offered a far from certain solution to the problem. Worse, it was still a new drug which in some patients had caused pain in the back, chills and vomiting, and in certain cases clinical shock.

There was talk of an antidote in development, but this was not yet available to Kolff. The third problem, yet to confront him, was the physical damage the kidney machine might do to the red blood cells.

With so many fundamental questions hanging over the operation of the machine, and doubtless with many more yet to present themselves, it might be argued that Kolff was foolhardy to proceed. It was common medical practice then to experiment on dogs before humans. Should he not have done the same? He remembers, with some relief, 'I never did an experiment on dogs or animals with the artificial kidney. That has been my salvation. I later learned that it is far more difficult to do in dogs than in human patients. If I had tried it first in animals, I would probably have given up.'

The first patient, although unrecorded in Kolff's papers, was an elderly Jew, Gustav Boele. You will not find his name in any medical records, and certainly not in Kolff's thesis. His was the forgotten dialysis. Extremely ill and confined to a hospital bed for many months, his sickness had prevented him from being transported to a Polish concentration camp with the rest of his family. Somehow he had been overlooked and officially he ceased to exist. The German authorities certainly knew nothing of his whereabouts, and the hospital was not going to tell them. In fact, Kolff had risked his own neck many times in order to treat Boele's many conditions, and the old man had now attained the status of the hospital's secret friend. He was suffering from a tumour of the prostate gland which had swollen to a size where it prevented urination, and he would die soon. His urine had backed up into the kidneys and caused uraemia, the treatment of which was Kolff's major ambition for his artificial kidney. Why not try the machine on old Boele?

Kolff had reservations as to whether his machine and techniques were sufficiently advanced, but the head nurse urged him to give it a go. 'She was an absolutely wonderful woman and said, "Why don't we try it? He's going to die anyway".' He was also anxious about how history might view his willingness to conduct what appeared to be an experiment on an elderly Jew. His conscience, he decided, was clear, for he had cared for Boele as well as for any other patient in the hospital with never a thought of discrimination. Kolff says, 'I had forgotten all about him until Janke reminded me of it. He was never published.' Forgotten in life, poor Boele was to be largely forgotten in death, too.

In the spirit of a rehearsal rather than a clinical experiment, Kolff decided he could draw a small quantity of the old man's blood, pass it through his newly constructed artificial kidney, and see what happened. There was little to lose. When Boele sank into a coma, his prognosis bleak, Kolff was persuaded it was the right thing to do, and the machine was made ready. The dialysing fluid was carefully measured out and mixed, and the sterilisation procedures commenced.

Janke had come to watch the first dialysis, although it wasn't his intention that she should stay. It went far from smoothly and the omens were not good. To begin with the old man's arteries proved so brittle that the insertion of a canula proved impossible, so Kolff was forced to remove only a small amount of blood, about 50 cc, from a vein in his arm. Dosed with heparin, this was passed into the cellophane tubing and the artificial kidney started to revolve, driven by a sewing-machine motor.

It soon became clear that all was not going to plan. The machine suffered numerous leaks, and when crimson foam started to appear in the dialysing bath it was obvious that blood was leaking from the cellophane tubing. The action of the ripples on the surface of the aluminium drum were having the effect of an egg whisk and turning the albumen in the blood into voluminous foam. Nevertheless Kolff was able to collect the blood which had successfully passed through the machine, and returned it to the old man's body via a vein in his arm. Even so, the scene could hardly have inspired confidence. The fluid in Berk's enamel tank had lapped over the edge, slopping around until the floor was awash with foam and blood. Shortly after that the struggling sewing-machine motor which was driving the drum failed. Janke stepped in and for fifteen minutes turned the artificial kidney by hand. Kolff decided they needed more help, and so Bob van Noordwijk was called for.

Despite this uncertain dialysis, bordering on a fiasco compared with his later efforts, Kolff felt some slight satisfaction. But the old man remained in a coma and Kolff admits it remains doubtful whether the dialysis of such a small quantity of blood, even if it were successful, had the slightest effect on his condition.

Kolff, throughout his career, was the first to admit failure, especially to fellow professionals. He knew it was vital to his work that he should have a good relationship with other doctors and specialists so that they might, with confidence, recommend suitable patients for treatment. That required considerable trust on their part, for Kolff's machine remained distinctly experimental. 'In Kampen, I organised a conference every week for doctors and physicians in the town. There were eight of them. Very soon, internists and other physicians from Groningen would also come, and professors would give lectures.' At those meetings, Kolff remembers, 'I always first admitted to my mistakes. It made it easier for the GPs.'

Nevertheless, despite his massaging of medical opinion, it was six months before Kolff was presented with his first suitable case for treatment. Had they not fully trusted him, or had for some inexplicable reason instances of kidney failure suddenly disappeared from north-east Holland? The wait was worth it, though, for the first patient sent to him filled Kolff's requirements precisely. It was his intention to use the artificial kidney only to provide what might be called temporary relief. Rather like a walking stick to aid a limping man, Kolff expected his artificial kidney to provide support to the natural kidneys until they could recover their full function and the artificial organ would be of no further use.

In Janny Schrijver Kolff saw an ideal patient for his first recorded dialysis. He remembers her as 'twenty-eight years old, not married, a housemaid and a nice woman'. She had felt increasingly ill, but had worked until she collapsed, and arrived by ambulance with her father, a peasant farmer, on 16 March 1943. She had initially been seen by an ophthalmologist, after complaining of deteriorating eyesight, and a doctor at the nearby hospital at Zwolle, who had diagnosed high blood pressure and chronic nephritis, a general term for inflammation of the kidneys. There were several possible causes. Her kidneys were rapidly failing, and like so many before her the prognosis was bleak and her condition poor. She complained of palpitations and a tightness in her chest, and her blood pressure was measured as very high at 245/150. But it was the urea level in her blood which posed the greatest threat, for the first analysis put it at 1.69 grams per litre (in a normal person a level of 0.3 grams per litre would be considered usual). As a consequence of the increasing failure of her kidneys to rid her blood of toxins, her sight was rapidly deteriorating, her mental processes were confused, her heart was racing. Kolff thought that at last he had a patient for whom he could provide temporary relief until her own kidneys recovered, and he agreed to try treatment with his artificial kidney. He attempted to explain the procedure to the young woman's father in the simplest possible terms, while at the same time making clear the risks. He said to him, 'Janny's blood is poisoned. We want to take part of the blood out of Janny's body, run it through a machine that will remove the poison, and return the blood to her body. You may stand by her if you like, and watch to see that nothing wrong is being done to her.' But when asked if he was certain of success, Kolff replied in all honesty that he could make no promises but would do his best. The father then suggested, 'Let the minister come first, after that you can try it.' The Revd Gastman duly made his call, the family prayed together, then Janny Schrijver was wheeled into Kolff's treatment room on a narrow bed built specially for kidney patients to negotiate the unusually narrow door.

Schrijver was unconscious when the preparation of the machine began. In his thesis Kolff described the procedure for sterilisation:

All parts of the artificial kidney coming into contact with blood, i.e. tubes, glasswork, rotation-couplings and bubble catcher, are cleaned so as to free them from all pyrogenic [fever-inducing] substances, and sterilised with the same care as that with which an apparatus for a blood transfusion is treated. Whether rigors occur or not is for the greater part dependent on this.

The tubes and the glass may be sterilised in an autoclave or boiled before dialysis, for which we had a big pan made. New cellophane is pyrogen free [unable to harbour organisms which might cause fever], and need only be rinsed and boiled, for which purpose it is wound on a wooden reel. We take a new cellophane tube for each dialysis. The other parts of the kidney, which do not come into direct contact with blood, must be clean, but need not be sterile. Cellophane is impermeable to bacteria and viruses. So the sterile cellophane tube can be seized with the hand. The water of the bath is not sterile either, and need not be so, if it is made up freshly.

Kolff proceeded with caution, and for the first dialysis took only half a litre of blood from Janny Schrijver, ran it through the machine, and gave it back to her. She regained consciousness and reported that she felt much better, but Kolff was not sure. 'The power of suggestion was enormous, but the dialysis of the first half litre of blood could not have done anything for her. Anyway, that was all we did on the first day, and then we waited twenty-four hours to see what happened next. Nothing happened, so we guessed it was safe to proceed.'

The extraction of the blood, and its return, was carefully monitored by van Noordwijk. It was a cumbersome procedure which involved the raising and lowering of a glass burette by a rope attached to a pulley on the ceiling. When the burette was lowered to below the level of the patient, a valve was opened to allow the patient's blood to flow into the burette. When Kolff decided sufficient had been collected, the valve was closed, cutting off the blood flow from the patient. Then van Noordwijk was given the signal to pull the string to raise the burette to the ceiling, then he opened another valve to allow the blood to flow into the cellophane tubing.

While the blood was passing through the tubing, he lowered the now empty burette from the ceiling so that it was ready to collect the blood as it emerged from the dialyser. When it had all been collected, the valve was closed to shut off the dialyser, then the burette was raised again to the ceiling, and the dialysed blood allowed to flow back into the patient. It was slow and tedious, dialysing cupful by cupful. But care had to be taken, for should positive pressure develop in the vein to which the blood was returned, the whole process might come to a sudden halt. It was van Noordwijk's job to make sure the return of the blood ran smoothly, and in order to monitor the level in the burette (which was now hoisted high up to the ceiling) he sat staring up at it with a pair of binoculars. What an increasingly bizarre sight it was becoming, Kolff and his team 'playing at kidneys'. Van Noordwijk remembers, 'We were all exhausted, tired by the excitement of it.' The slightest tear in the cellophane and the blood would leak into the dialysing tank, resulting in that rising tide of crimson foam to which they were becoming increasingly accustomed. Kolff noted in his records, 'Our motto was that there was nothing to be lost and perhaps a temporary improvement to be gained.'

The first dialysis, van Noordwijk remembers, took only 22 minutes, but it was to be the first of many carried out on Janny Schrijver, and Kolff was convinced that his patient was well able to survive the procedure. In all, she was dialysed twelve times in as many days, and by the tenth dialysis the procedure lasted no less than six hours. By this stage she was undoubtedly in a more relaxed mental state and vomited less. Kolff must have been increasingly hopeful, especially as the condition of his patient appeared to improve. At the same time the blackboard was becoming covered with increasingly optimistic figures as a result of the work of Mieneke van der Leij and Willy Eskes working long hours under enormous pressure to analyse samples of blood before and after dialysis.

Kolff became quietly confident. 'It was quite clear the machine was working. I knew all along that I wanted to remove urea, and I'd achieved that. I also measured all the other things we were removing from the blood: the creatinine, uric acid, and the electrolytes. The machine *was* working.'

Janny Schrijver, however, remained extremely sick and suffered from complications other than those attributable to her failing kidneys. The dose of heparin given by Kolff to prevent her blood clotting was massive – ten times the modern recommended dose – and she suffered chills and fevers as a result. The removal of the canula from the artery was made difficult by the inability of her blood to clot, and van Noordwijk remembers that the seventh dialysis 'caused very persistent haemorrhage'.

Kolff went on. 'We eventually took 12 litres of blood and ran it through the machine, then for the first time you could see the blood urea of the patient, which had been going up, had a dip before going up again. So I took 20 litres of blood, and that achieved a real dip. We had learned that we could do that without killing the patient, that was the important thing.'

Subsequent attempts at dialysis, however, became increasingly difficult. New needles were not available in wartime Holland, and the few Kolff had access to had been resharpened many times after sterilisation. Janny Schrijver herself was running out of blood vessels from which Kolff could draw blood. The options were rapidly running out.

Yet Kolff had proved that his machine worked: the urea level in her blood had stabilised, and her blood pressure had begun to fall. For fourteen days her uraemia did not worsen, even if her overall condition was complicated by heart failure and a multitude of infections. It was therefore Kolff's brave decision to connect the woman directly to the machine; instead of drawing off blood and returning it to her little by little, her entire bloodstream would be allowed to pass through the machine uninterrupted.

Van Noordwijk remembers those long dialyses as being

hypnotic affairs, always conducted at night so that they didn't interfere with the running of the hospital, and Kolff could give them his undivided attention. 'The revolving of the drum sounded like a waterwheel, and there was a rhythmic hum from the paddle which kept the dialysing fluid in motion. I once went to sleep for an hour in another room and on returning woke up to find the cellophane had broken, but no one had noticed.'

After the fourth dialysis Janny Schrijver recovered somewhat and spoke lucidly about her home and held conversations with the people round her bed. But the hoped-for improvement in the natural function of her kidneys, which Kolff believed might take place if his machine relieved them of their burden, failed to happen. After two days of no dialysis, the results from Kolff's laboratory showed her urea levels were climbing fast and she would soon return to a comatose state. He dialysed twice with increased urgency.

On the twenty-sixth day, his patient having lived almost a month longer because of his treatment, Kolff was forced to admit defeat. Yet it was not his inability to dialyse her that stopped him. He had simply run out of veins and arteries to which he could make a connection. She was taken back to the ward, as Kolff was unable to help her further. Soon the laboratory showed the urea level in her blood was rising fast. Shortly after, the world's first patient to experience continuous kidney dialysis died, on 4 May.

Her father came to the hospital to collect the body and called on Kolff to thank him for his efforts. He asked how much he should pay? Kolff tried to waive any suggestion of money, but the old man insisted. 'I felt he would be much happier if he could pay me something', Kolff remembers. 'I charged him sixty guilders. Dialysis need not be expensive. I thought then that you could set up an artificial kidney

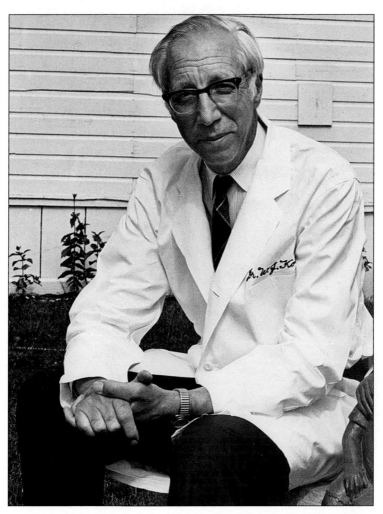

Willem Johann Kolff, inventor of the world's first kidney machine, seen here when Head of the Division of Artificial Organs at the University of Utah in 1971. (*Willem Kolff collection*)

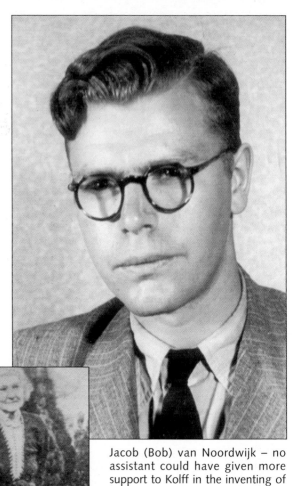

Jacob (Bob) van Noordwijk – no assistant could have given more support to Kolff in the inventing of the artificial kidney. (*Willem Kolff collection*)

Sofia Schafstadt – the pioneering patient. She was the first person whose life was undoubtedly saved by Kolff's artificial kidney. (*Willem Kolff collection*)

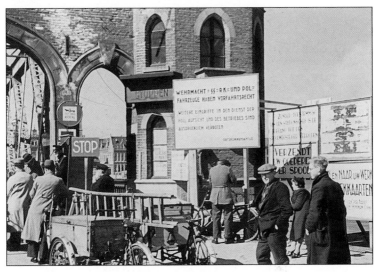

The Nazi occupiers in Kampen making life difficult at the bridge across the River Ijssel. (*Frans Walkate Archief*)

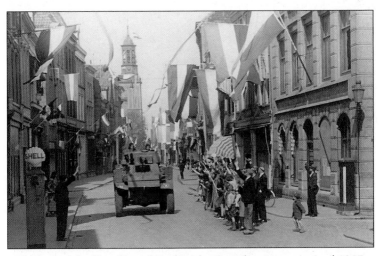

The longed-for liberation of Kampen by Canadian troops in April 1945, though some of the bleakest days were yet to come.
(*Frans Walkate Archief*)

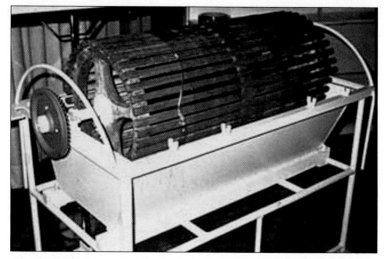

One of Kollf's first artificial kidneys, 1946. Precious kidney machines were sent to medical centres around the world, including the comparative post-war safety of Edinburgh, London, New York, Poland and Montreal. (*Royal Infirmary, Edinburgh*)

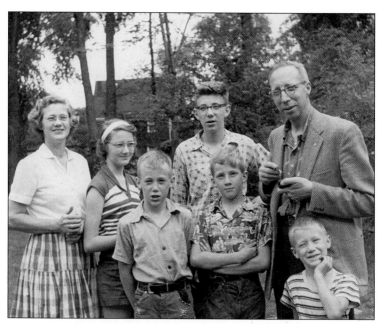

By 1954, the Kolffs were well settled in America. From left to right: Janke, Adrie, Albert, Jack, Kees, Pim, Therus. (*Willem Kolff*)

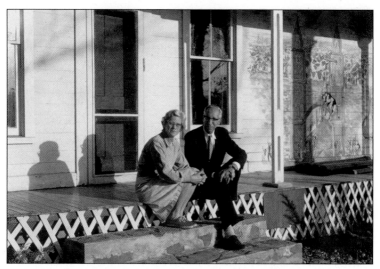

Janke and Pim Kolff sit on the steps of the Cleveland farmhouse – an escape from the professional pressures of the Clinic. The mural, depicting Kampen, suggests that a little of their hearts remained in the Netherlands. (*Willem Kolff*)

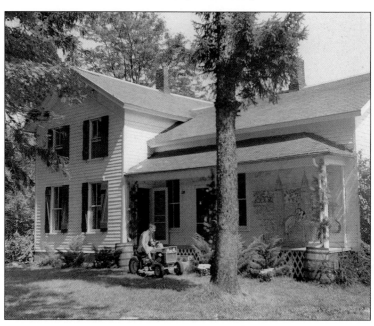

Money was in short supply: some of the rooms in the farmhouse were furnished with discarded hospital beds. (*Willem Kolff*)

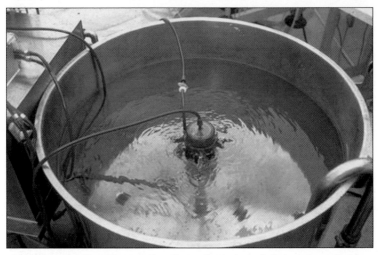

Much simpler than the rotating drum: the twin-coil dialyser invented by Kolff and Watschinger. (*Royal Infirmary, Edinburgh*)

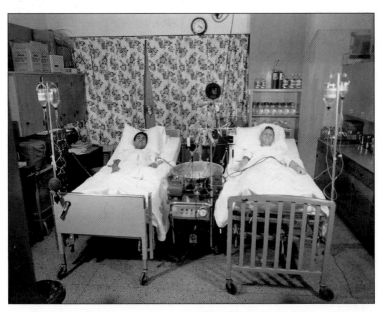

The twin-coil kidney made in 1955 by Kolff and Watschinger. Two patients are shown sharing the same bath. (*Special Collections Dept, J. Willard Marriott Library, University of Utah*)

Dialysis machines need not be expensive: Kolff, centre, inspects an early home dialyser prototype, using a washing machine as a dialysing tank – much to the distress of the Maytag company. To the left is Dr Satoru Nakamoto, to the right Dr Yuki Nose. (*From Paul I. Terasaki (ed.),* History of Transplantation: 35 Recollections, *The UCLA Tissue Typing Laboratory, 1991*)

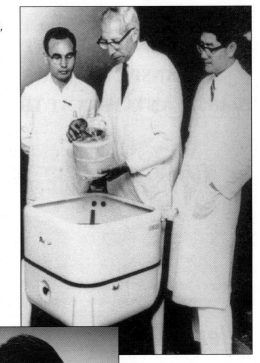

Dr Robert Jarvik holds the Jarvik-7 artificial heart. Dr Barney Clark was the first to undergo such an operation, on 1 December 1982 at the University of Utah Medical Center, Salt Lake City. (*Hank Morgan/Science Photo Library*)

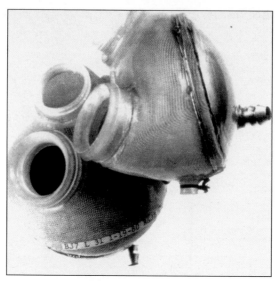

An early artificial heart from Kolff's laboratory carrying the name of its principal designer, Jarvik. (*ICMT (International Center for Medical Technologies) Archive, with permission*)

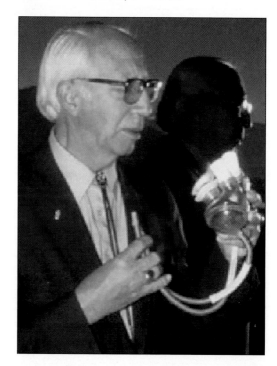

Dr Willem Kolff with the artificial heart which he and Robert Jarvik developed. (*ICMT (International Center for Medical Technologies) Archive, with permission*)

very cheaply. All you needed was tap water, sausage skin and some sterilising fluid, then go ahead.'

Indeed, the quest for cheap and ready dialysis was to occupy many of his thoughts in years to come. But in the meantime he recorded for publication the details of the treatment Janny Schrijver had undergone: 'I have noted carefully everything that went wrong so that others would learn from the experience. This has always been my principle.' If the death of Schrijver depressed him, he didn't show it. Instead, he ordered the building of a second kidney machine, larger than the first, in the increasingly firm belief that one day his apparatus would save lives.

6
A MACHINE OF LAST RESORT

In the short time since Berk had built the first kidney machine, much had changed in the wartime atmosphere of Kampen, making Kolff's job ever more difficult. The Kampen Enamel Works came under ever closer scrutiny from the Germans and it was unlikely that any more dawn meetings would go unnoticed, and certainly the construction of a medical machine would not go unspotted by the increasingly vigilant Germans. Berk agreed to make the enamel bath, but Kolff would have to look elsewhere for the rest of the apparatus.

With aluminium now in short supply, Kolff returned to the materials he knew best from his childhood days. At the carpenter's bench in his father's sanatorium, when only six years old, he had learned the virtues and versatility of wood, and so when Berk declined to build another machine on the grounds that it was no longer safe for him to do so, and anyway he had little metal to spare, Kolff turned to the local wheelwright, whose everyday job was the repair of farm carts and wagons. As a consequence the second machine had rather an agricultural look about it and less of the engineering gloss which Berk would have given it. The slats around which the cellophane tubing was wrapped were made out of beech, and the dialysing tank was held in place by a wooden frame, probably made of ash, which would have been a wheelwright's preferred material.

This change in the method of construction, in building the laths out of wood and not of metal, had one important consequence, as Bob van Noordwijk remembers: 'The rotation of the drum in the water no longer caused a soft rustling as the first kidney did, but instead it made a clear splashing. This was muffled when there was a leak in the tubing, causing clouds of foam to overflow the rim of the tank and on to the floor.'

When the second kidney machine had been delivered to Kampen Hospital, the first became free and was dispatched to The Hague and set up in the hospital where Kolff had established the first blood bank in mainland Europe back in 1940. Bob van Noordwijk delivered it in a small van, and was indignant at the reception he got. He remembers, 'I arrived at the hospital and informed the porter, as if it were the most common thing in the world, that I had come to deliver an artificial kidney machine. His reaction surprised me. "From which firm are you coming to give a demonstration?" I was indignant. Just imagine, I had not come to *sell* something, but to help the hospital set up an important medical invention. But, of course, the porter couldn't be expected to know this.'

The indifferent porter spoke unwittingly for many in the medical world when he asked about what machine, what's the importance of it, what are you trying to sell us? Few people other than Kolff and his close associates were yet ready to believe it represented any sort of a breakthrough. Indeed, when the new machine performed its first dialysis in Kampen, the results were again less than encouraging from the point of view of saving life. The sixty-year-old patient, suffering from renal tuberculosis, had indeed improved in condition shortly after treatment, as Janny Schrijver had, and started to pass increasing amounts of urine, indicating some improvement in the functioning of his kidneys. But as Kolff's notes record, 'The pains in his bladder were of such a nature that we believed we had no right to prolong this man's life any further.' The machine over which so many questions hovered had still not been proved to be a life-saver.

The original kidney machine stood for some months in the hospital at The Hague awaiting a suitable patient, and it wasn't until November 1943 that Dr Holmer of the department of medicine thought he had an ideal case. The man was suffering from acute glomerulonephritis (a group of diseases that affect the glomeruli which are at the heart of the kidney's filtration mechanisms). Over a period of two weeks he had passed less and less urine but was thought well enough by doctors in The Hague to undergo treatment with Kolff's radical machine. Curiosity must also have played a part, for a large part of the staff watched as van Noordwijk made meticulous adjustments to the machine while Kolff prepared the patient.

Unfortunately the patient proved to be less well than was at first thought. When the time came for dialysis, he had already suffered a temporary cessation of breathing and was almost comatose by the time he was connected to the artificial kidney. The motor was switched on, the dialyser came to life and the long, slow treatment began. It restored little life to the poor patient. Having removed no less than 80 grams of urea in the course of a seven-hour dialysis with little obvious improvement in his condition, it was agreed there was no point in prolonging his treatment, and he died shortly after the kidney was disconnected. Nevertheless the attempt had helped to spread the reputation of the machine, for now it had been demonstrated to a wider audience that it was capable of performing the cleansing functions of a natural kidney. The remaining major hurdle of saving a life had yet to be jumped.

The original kidney machine soon found itself on the move once again, this time to an emergency hospital set up in a converted school in Amsterdam, near the Vondel Park.

When the time came to attempt the first dialysis here, Kolff and van Noordwijk travelled from Kampen to operate the machine and supervise the treatment, but the emergency hospital did not have the sterilising equipment needed to fully cleanse the rubber and glass tubes, the connecting pieces or the cellophane. Van Noordwijk parcelled everything together, put it under his arm and took a tram heading towards the Central Laboratory of the Red Cross Blood Transfusion Service, where he was able to sterilise everything using high pressure steam equipment. He remembers, 'The atmosphere was tense in Amsterdam at the time. The strike of May 1943 had only just ended and the air was alive with rumours of new round-ups by the Germans. However, I never came across a problem; even so I preferred to stay on the rear, open balcony of the tram with the parts of the artificial kidney under my arm, just in case I had to make a quick exit.' He needn't have taken the risk. The patient's kidney function had returned naturally and no dialysis was performed that night.

This was an increasingly difficult time throughout Holland as food and fuel were in ever shorter supply, and it was at no small personal risk that Kolff and van Noordwijk travelled the country to operate their kidney machine. In April 1943 the supreme commander of the German troops in Holland, General Christiansen, announced that 300,000 former members of the Dutch armed forces were to report for internment in Germany. The Third Reich was now under increasing pressure. Having failed to capture Stalingrad, 94,000 German troops had surrendered to the Russians after their first major defeat of the war, and Hitler had upped the stakes by declaring that Germany was in a state of 'total war'. This meant a merciless tightening of the regimes in occupied countries. The Netherlands felt the Nazi grip like never before. With its increasing military commitments,

Germany became short of manpower, particularly in the armaments factories, and although women had been called in to help there were too few of them to make any real impact. The Nazi eye turned towards the Dutch labour force. Many Dutchmen had already refused to set foot in Germany – this time they would not be allowed the luxury of choice.

The conscription of Dutch army veterans produced outrage, and as a result armament workers in Hengelo, in eastern Holland, came out on strike. They were joined by other workers in the town and the strike quickly spread until groups as far apart as the coal miners of Limburg and the Philips workers in Eindhoven had joined. Farm workers in the area around Kampen also supported the protest, until half a million workers were on strike.

The Germans reacted by announcing a 'police state of siege' and warnings were given that anyone who disobeyed the order to return to work would be shot. In the sense that most took that warning seriously and dutifully returned to work, the strike was lost. But in reminding the Germans that the Dutch would have nothing to do with the Nazi cause, and that even in defeat they were not a pushover, the strike was without doubt important. Yet against this background of threatened executions, of public shootings and civil unrest, young van Noordwijk and Kolff walked the streets of Holland with their precious brown paper parcels of rubber tubing and sausage skins, determined to save life.

In the autumn of that year a third kidney machine was built which was taken by van Noordwijk by boat from Kampen to Amsterdam, where it was to be housed in the blood transfusion centre in the care of Dr Spaander. Meanwhile, in Kampen, Kolff had conducted yet another unsuccessful treatment on a 68-year-old man suffering from cancer of the kidneys. The man was in shock and his circulation in a poor state even before the treatment started. It was a blatantly hopeless case. The dialysis was stopped and the patient soon died. Kolff's next patient, again a 68-year-old man, had come to Kampen Hospital for treatment for a hernia which had resulted in infection. He became very ill, drowsy and uraemic after five days, and by the time he was brought to Kolff he was verging on comatose. Remarkably, after his dialysis he woke up and spoke with his family. But his grasp on life was slender and he was recorded as having 'lost breath and died'.

The sixth attempt at dialysis took place in Amsterdam. Spaander had promised Kolff he would make contact as soon as he had a suitable patient available, and when the call finally came through Kolff and van Noordwijk headed for Amsterdam on one of the few trains still running. There they found the kidney machine had been set up in a disused room in the emergency hospital. The patient was Greta Cleef, a young woman aged thirty-three. Although she recovered from a bout of scarlet fever, she had been left with acute nephritis. Kolff measured the urea level in her blood. It was very high: 5.3 grams per litre. She slipped into unconsciousness.

Van Noordwijk started to prepare the machine. This was the start of a process which was going to take thirty hours, throughout all of which Kolff was to remain on duty and awake. However, his first problem was of a mechanical and not a medical nature. It was a problem which had already presented itself in Kampen and was entirely due to the fact that Kolff's artificial kidney machines had, of necessity, been set up in rooms that were unused at the time. They were neither hospital wards nor operating theatres – and the doors were not designed to accommodate a hospital bed. As Greta Cleef was wheeled down the corridor to the kidney machine, it soon became apparent that the bed would not go through the door. Kolff recorded in a matter of fact way in his notes: 'In those days my doctor's bag did contain electrician's pliers and a set of screwdrivers, but no crowbar.' Those few tools, however, were sufficient for a little rebuilding of the doorway by Kolff before the dialysis could commence.

There followed a marathon seventeen-hour dialysis. During those long hours, his mind doubtless dulled by the hypnotic splashing as the laths dipped in and out of the dialysing tank, Kolff remained sufficiently alert to make a remarkable observation – his patient started to shrink before his eyes. At first he couldn't believe what he was seeing. What was happening was that Cleef's body, unable to secrete surplus fluid owing to the failure of her kidneys, had become bloated through oedema. But while she was connected to the artificial kidney, the excess fluids were being removed at such a rate that the woman's swollen hands shrank visibly while Kolff watched. The full potency of his machine was now brought home to him.

It made the machine a highly dangerous piece of equipment, for the damage done to the body by the rapid removal of such huge quantities of fluid could have had catastrophic results. On his own admission Kolff had been lucky. Thinking that the machine might do physical damage to the red blood cells, he had employed a technique he had learned while setting up his blood bank, and added glucose to the dialysing fluid. As Kolff explains, 'In my original kidney, the blood is under no pressure so to remove the excess water I added glucose to the dialysing fluid. This would create the right conditions for the excess water to pass through the membrane and out of the blood. Without my knowing it, this saved me a lot of trouble. If you are removing urea quickly from the blood, and remember you might be taking out the equivalent of a jam jar full of the stuff, you get quick and sudden changes in the balances of the electrolytes in the blood and it takes time for them to settle. Until they come right, you can get a disequilibrium syndrome which can make the patient very ill. High glucose in the bloodstream prevents that. I cannot prove it, but that is what I think happened. If I hadn't used glucose, patients would have died from that disequilibrium and I would not have known why. It was very lucky that we used glucose.'

After ten hours Greta Cleef woke, and by the morning was fully conscious and able to talk in a coherent way about her family. Kolff must have felt deeply optimistic at the result, especially when her own kidneys started to excrete urine, proving that some natural recovery was taking place. It looked as though he was on the verge of his first triumph, and he thought how sad it would be if his gang of supporters who had kept faith with him through all the early disappointments were not there to see it. Sadly, the atmosphere of optimism was soon shattered. Within twenty-four hours the woman developed a raging fever and died swiftly of pneumonia. Kolff too was almost dead on his feet.

His self-belief never left him for long, however. He had a growing suspicion that patients were dying not through any failing in his machine but because they were going to die anyway. Only when they were deeply ill, so sick that they were almost dead, were the doctors sending them to him. Instead of being their last resort, he wanted to be their first, and on returning to Kampen he wasted no time in reminding the medical community that he needed kidney patients who had only recently become ill, instead of those who were beyond any kind of help. One former assistant of Kolff's remarked, 'The doctors did not send people until they were dying on the theory that, although Kolff could not help them, at least he could no longer harm them.'

The delay in sending patients to him caused all kinds of needless complications. Those in an advanced stage of kidney failure were found to have fragile blood vessels hardly able to stand simple surgery, like the insertion of the necessary tubes. (Even the tubes themselves became scarce when all rubber piping was requisitioned by the German army.) Those who remember the early days of dialysis say that Kolff's spirits fell as often as they rose. It was not uncommon for him to remain at the hospital all night, surviving on tea and anything his troubled stomach could tolerate. On one occasion Kolff had invited along members of the local medical establishment to view for themselves the operation of his kidney machine, but the delicate cellophane tubing burst and the patient's blood seeped into the dialysing tank, resulting in the inevitable crimson foam which was always the harbinger of bad news about the way the dialysis was proceeding. Those Kolff sought to impress went away from Kampen Hospital concerned rather than persuaded by Kolff's experiments. A colleague remembers that such disasters caused him profound gloom. He might cycle home forgetting to remove his surgical mask, and wonder why everyone on the street stared at him as he cycled by.

But there was always the prospect of the next patient, the one for whom dialysis would prove to be a life-saver. If Kolff himself could have had the choice, he would have selected a patient suffering from an infection or inflammation of the kidneys which had caused a temporary loss of function. The condition would have been only recently diagnosed, so that complications would not have already set in. Then the machine could provide relief and aid a recovery of natural function. There was no suggestion at this time that dialysis would be a regular procedure, carried out every three days for the rest of the patient's life. Kolff knew that there was a limit to the number of times the connections could be made to the patient's body before he ran out of access veins or arteries, since entry points could not be reused.

Then word of yet another potential patient came through, and on the basis of the description given, he sounded ideal. Galvanised with a new enthusiasm and suffused with optimism once again, van Noordwijk was asked to set up the kidney machine and the laboratory technicians were put on standby for yet another long night's work. Dialyses were usually carried out at night. Kolff explained, 'I was too damned busy. I had to make a living. It wasn't because I was afraid the Germans would see what I was up to, it was simply because that was the only time available.'

The patient, called Termeulen, was a young, fat man who worked as a baker. To Kolff's disappointment, he was almost dead when he arrived at the hospital. The urea level in his blood was a deadly 7 grams. The only thing that persuaded Kolff to proceed was that this was a case of acute kidney failure which had come over the baker suddenly, and so it was possible that the patient would have a chance of recovery if Kolff could take over the function of his natural kidneys for a while.

The preparations were by now becoming well rehearsed and almost routine. If the set-up procedure changed it was due to shortages of piping, needles, connectors or cellophane tubing. The blackboard was wiped clean and made ready for the new analyses at which Kolff's laboratory was now well practised. His army was on top fighting form, and more than ready to score a victory.

Termeulen's dialysis lasted fourteen long hours, until all his blood had been through the machine no fewer than twenty-four times. The quantity of urea extracted was impressive, and if dried and returned to crystalline form would have filled a sugar bowl. It was going well. Then Termeulen woke. Even better news – he asked for a newspaper.

Three days later the young man was still alive, but blood tests showed the urea was again accumulating in his blood, even though there was some positive evidence that his kidneys had resumed something of their normal function. In fact, hour by hour the volume of excreted urine rose, which was yet another sign that his natural kidney function was returning. Spirits rose accordingly.

Three days later the most promising patient so far died. If he had been sent to him sooner, Kolff believed, he might have stood a chance. The patients were still coming to him 'too *damned* late'. Termeulen was yet another failure to add to the ever lengthening list.

It is a mark of Kolff's single-minded determination that he never gave up. He said, 'I start to feel unhappy and discontented if I think about disappointment. But I was always very unhappy when I lost a patient. Several days before he dies, I often think he recognises the inevitability and then he cries, sometimes with joy. I was always very involved, and had an acute sense of what my patients were going through.'

To read the outcome of the dialyses on the first fifteen patients, though, would depress even the most optimistic of souls. It is a sad list of repeated failure despite heroic struggle, but failure nevertheless. Kolff's notes read:

Patient 7 . . . was treated twice with the artificial kidney but died of the consequences of a staphylococcal infection [penicillin was not yet known] which had caused his kidney problem in the first place. Patient 8 . . . the dialysis was terminated prematurely because the patient's general condition became so bad that it was useless to carry on. Patient 9 . . . the patient died the day after dialysis. [Patient 10 survived the dialysis and recovered, but it was thought that this was little to do with the effects of the dialysis and so Kolff could claim no success here.] Patient 11 . . . the blood pressure remained high. He died of cardiac failure four days after the dialysis. Patient 14 . . . he survived dialysis for only a few hours. Patient 16 . . . two days later he died, just before he was going to be connected to the kidney for the second time.

Despite the loss of life, Kolff's machine was stunningly successful at replicating the effects of the human kidney. He had by now been able to measure its efficiency scientifically and compare it with the workings of the human kidney, and calculated, for example, that the total length of the filtration membranes in a human kidney was no less than 75 kilometres, whereas in his kidney the cellophane tube was less than 45 metres long. And whereas he calculated the quantity of blood purified in the human kidney per minute at about 70 cc, his machine processed over double that, even though only 150 cc of blood per minute flowed through the cellophane tubing, whereas the human kidney demanded 1.5 litres. In other words this was an extraordinarily efficient dialyser. Not only did it perform the functions of the human kidney, it was *better* at them. Even if development went no further, it was already a remarkable achievement.

Not that Kolff was satisfied. Neither was Berk, the enamel maker who had helped construct the first machine, and who was reported to be very depressed at the loss of life of those connected to the machine. After hearing the lengthening list of fatalities, he told friends that he wished he'd never had anything to do with it.

7

A MISERABLE CONVOY OF MEN AND BOYS

The spring and summer of 1944 in the Netherlands was no time to be working on medical breakthroughs; survival in increasingly harsh conditions was work enough for Kampen Hospital. A fourth Kolff child, Albert, was born in June 1944 to add further to the pressures of feeding an ever-growing family and keeping it cheerful in a wartime atmosphere.

The hardship suffered by the people of Kampen was acute, as it was throughout much of the Netherlands. To everyone, it seemed that the greater the pressure on the Germans as the Allies fought back, the less tolerable life became as the Germans progressively robbed the Dutch of their workforce, and even the food from their fields. The liberation of the province of Limburg at the beginning of September had added to the hardship, as this was the only source of coal in the Netherlands, and those living north of the Rhine had access to no other fuel.

With an acute sense of when trouble was brewing, and through impeccable contacts in the resistance, Kolff knew when it was time for him and his team to keep their heads down. He was especially protective of young van Noordwijk, so that the young man who had already fallen foul of the Germans once should not do so again. Van Noordwijk remembers, 'Kolff would say to me, "I expect there will be trouble shortly; you'd better go away for a few days." Of course, I did not ask why: it had become second nature not to react with questions to such warnings, for if you did not know anything you could not be forced to confess to it if you were arrested by the Germans. So I left Kampen and stayed with the parents of one of my friends who had gone underground because he refused to sign a declaration of allegiance to the German authorities, which all university students were compelled to sign in order to continue their studies.' It was decades later that Kolff explained why he had asked his assistant to leave so urgently on one occasion: it was the day before the planned assassination of the chief of police.

Nevertheless, in early September 1944 there was a glimmer of hope that the war in the Netherlands might be coming to an end. The Dutch had been watching the Allies' steady advance northwards since the liberation of Paris. Montgomery's tanks has pushed north with ease against a disorganised German Army, and by 4 September had reached the Belgian city of Antwerp. Dutch hopes grew higher as German fears increased, resulting in a day well remembered in Holland as 'Dolle Dinsdag' – Mad Tuesday – as the German army fled north and east through Holland. Their flight caused much rejoicing. Surely this was a sign that the war would be over soon.

Disappointment was quick to follow. Although they did not know it then, for many Dutch the most cruel phase of the war was about to begin. Allied supply lines had been unable to match the rapid advance northwards, which had met with surprisingly little opposition. It gave the Germans the opportunity they needed to regroup and establish a new front. After a brief burst of optimism, the Dutch found themselves back at square one.

Kolff issued another warning to Bob van Noordwijk, possibly his most stern yet, in mid-September 1944. 'Bob, I expect trouble here. You'd better disappear. Go to my father's sanatorium in Beekbergen.' A sanatorium was a relatively safe place, for German troops were so scared of tuberculosis that they kept away from anywhere it might be present. Without question, Bob packed a few things and cycled off. On the way he was warned that the Germans were rounding up men near Apeldoorn, so he took a side road and arrived safely in Beekbergen. It was here, on the morning of 17 September, that he woke to the sound of gunfire – the opening shots in Operation Market Garden.

This was an audacious attempt by the Allies to secure the bridges across the Dutch rivers to enable them to advance rapidly into the industrial regions of Germany, avoiding the Siegfried Line (which was Germany's primary protection). Had the operation been successful, the war would undoubtedly have been over by Christmas 1944. To coincide with, and bolster, the operation, the Dutch government in exile called for a strike of the Dutch railway workers to hinder further the Germans' ability to move troops, ammunition and reinforcements. It required courage for a Dutch railway worker to go on strike, for such action would undoubtedly be considered as giving aid to the Allies – for which the penalty, if caught, was certain death.

Van Noordwijk decided he would spent the rest of the war in Groningen, and planned to cycle there, hiding one night in a haystack when word reached him of yet another round-up of able-bodied men by the Germans. After discussions with Kolff, it was decided that it was unsafe for a young man already convicted of anti-German activities to stay in Kampen. His departure was not simple, however, for the bridge crossing the River Ijssel was closely guarded, except on Thursdays, which was market day. That was when van Noordwijk made his escape. A couple of days later he was in Groningen and went into hiding for the rest of the war. Kolff had lost a staunch supporter. Meanwhile less than 100 miles from Kampen the battle for control of the bridge at Arnhem had ended in failure for the Allies after ten days of ferocious fighting. As Lieutenant-General Browning famously remarked of the campaign, 'I think we might be going a bridge too far.'

For Kolff, thoughts of further work on the artificial kidney became an ambition too far. It was difficult even to find transport to bring severely ill patients into hospital for established treatment, let alone think about the possibility of finding suitable patients for Kolff's kidney machine. He had also lost his clinical technician, van Noordwijk.

Suddenly it didn't matter. An all-eclipsing catastrophe was about to descend on the city of Kampen, and Kolff and the entire staff of Kampen Hospital were to be at the heart of it, all their energies directed to a life-saving operation on a vast scale.

Under increasing pressure, the Nazis decided that the men and boys of Rotterdam were an easy source of labour. In Germany they could be put to work digging trenches and building fortifications, and even pressed to fight for the Germans if they were old enough – a loathsome notion to a loyal Dutchman. Rotterdam was divided into blocks, and pamphlets were delivered to every house with the warning that all men between the ages of fifteen and forty-five, healthy or not, had to stand at their front door at eight o'clock the next morning with a spoon, a fork and sufficient food for four days. The Germans threatened that every house would be searched and any man found hiding would be immediately shot and a grenade thrown into the house – no arguments. To prove they meant it, a few Dutchmen were randomly shot and their bodies paraded on the street corners as a reminder. One effect of this mass round-up was that the Jews, many of whom had been in hiding for almost four years, not only risked their own lives if they remained in concealment, but also threatened the safety of their hosts who had risked much to give them shelter in the first place.

On what Kolff remembers as a 'miserable, wet day in Holland', the entire male population of Rotterdam was herded, like cattle, into the city's football stadium. The look of defeat on their faces can only be imagined. But the Nazi plan was running into trouble. An Allied bombardment of roads and bridges made transportation almost impossible, and what was left of Holland's transport system was already grinding to a halt. With no other option remaining, the Nazis resorted to using a fleet of barges to carry their prisoners to Germany and loaded eight thousand miserable souls on to beds of straw laid thickly in the bottom of the open craft. Ten of these barges left Rotterdam in convoy, bound north through the Ijsselmeer and then eastwards to the mouth of the Ijssel river; this would lead, eventually, to the Rhine. At the mouth of the Ijssel, of course, stood the city of Kampen.

As the hideous fleet of barges sailed into view, Kampen was presented with the most miserable convoy imaginable. Sick and able-bodied men and boys were packed into the barges, bedded on straw like livestock, bound for the German labour camps. The first man to recognise the full horror of what was happening was a local general practitioner, Dr Pel, who lived on Kampen quayside and was among the first to see the barges and their pathetic cargo as they approached the town. News quickly spread of the convoy of thousands of dispirited, sick and bewildered people that was about to descend on the city. Dr Pel called Kolff, urging him that something must be done.

'There were ten of these barges,' Kolff remembers, 'with 8,000 men in all, and among them were diabetics who had no insulin. There were several that were paralysed, there were the deaf and blind, and people with urinary containers. There were all kinds because they had been told to stand at their front doors whether they were sick or not.'

They were unceremoniously landed at Kampen and placed in the barracks that had once housed the Dutch Army. Now empty, the barracks were an abiding emblem to the people of Kampen of their army's defeat – a defeat which the arrival of the deportees only served to underline.

'They were busy unloading these people,' remembers Kolff, 'so I went to see the German commander and introduced myself. He was drunk, not very drunk but he had clearly been drinking. I said to him "these people are sick and of no use to you. If you like I will take them and put them into emergency hospitals and take care of them." I told him that many had influenza and pneumonia and some of them would die. Baatz, the German commander, then asked, "But what happens if they run away? Who will be responsible?" I told him I would be responsible. So he did a deal and said to me, "OK. If any of them run away, I will have *you* shot. How about that?" I said, "That's fine. Let's do it."'

Working with the local branch of the Red Cross, the local doctors and Dr Kehrer, the director of the hospital, Kolff established emergency hospitals in every available corner of Kampen. They pressed into service an empty orphanage and a large furniture factory on the far side of the river which had the advantage of holding a stock of timber out of which beds could be made. The evacuees themselves were far from useless; they proved to be a valuable resource, for among them were administrators who helped to devise a management system, in particular a card index with the name of every patient and his diagnosis. These records were cleverly devised in such a way that they could be easily falsified. The danger, of course, was that the round-up in Rotterdam had been so thorough and wide-ranging that it was possible, if not likely, that among them would have been Nazi sympathisers. 'We had to be careful because we could be betrayed at any moment if we put a foot wrong', says Kolff.

Every morning Kolff was required to present himself to the Nazi commander, Baatz, and deliver a list of his patients. It usually ran to about 350 names. On one occasion, while Kolff waited for Baatz's signature, he remembers overhearing him on the telephone, boasting to a superior officer that he had found a Jew in one of the barges, Abraham van der Schoot, and made him stand on the edge while he shot him. With great glee, Baatz described how the body fell into the river and was never seen again. Kolff wondered if he was merely boasting to prove to his commander what a strong and loyal soldier he was. However, it was later learned that he *had* shot the Jew.

Baatz was not Kolff's greatest enemy in Kampen, though. The mayor, a National Socialist appointed by the Germans in 1942, 'a real vile guy', was a far greater danger to Kolff. Baatz, after all, was merely obeying orders, whereas Mayor Sandberg had a wicked streak which the war had allowed him to fully exploit. Sandberg was convinced that Kolff was deceiving the authorities and that not all the people he and the other doctors were treating were genuinely ill. His suspicions may have been founded on fact, but it gave him the opportunity to exact his revenge for the refusal of Kampen Hospital to recognise his authority. He had been snubbed at every opportunity. Now they were to pay for their insolence. Sandberg urged the Germans to keep a careful eye on Kolff and to trust nothing that was happening in these makeshift hospitals.

For the first time during the war Kolff needed the help of the Germans. Only they could protect him from the inquisitive Sandberg. He also needed to be on closer terms with Baatz, to learn in advance of any plans for a surprise raid on his hospitals. 'Baatz had an eye for a very attractive Dutch girl with one of the most beautiful figures I have ever set my eyes on. Her fiancé had been deported to Germany and she wanted him back, so she befriended Baatz at every opportunity. That girl was very useful to me, and without her help I would often have been in great trouble. She was able to tell me everything that was going on, and as soon as they had made a plan for a surprise raid on the hospital, I knew when it was going to happen.'

Kolff's tactic turned from concealment to blatant exposure of his patients to Nazi inspection. Warned of an imminent raid by the loyal Dutch girl who had learned about it from Baatz, Kolff immediately dispatched an official invitation to the Germans to visit his patients. 'If you are correct and polite to Germans there is not usually a problem.' The Germans accepted, and a tour of the hospitals soon began.

A rearrangement of the patients had meanwhile taken place. In one large room in the old orphanage numerous epileptics, some of them hysterical, had been gathered. 'I was standing there with this German with his big uniform and his big boots, a massive guy, and a patient in one of the beds nearest us started to convulse. So violent was the thrashing that a Red Cross girl came with pillows to make sure he didn't hurt himself against the iron bedstead. Then another started to have a violent fit, which set another off, then another until it was like bedlam in that room. The German said, "Let's get out of here", and that was the end of the inspection. To make sure we got no more trouble from that German, I'd arranged with a local merchant to have some Dutch gin, and I gave him a good glass of it. I never had any more trouble from him.'

Kolff had been even more cunning than it first appears, for during the course of the hospital inspection he had pointed out to the Germans that the apparatus standing in the corner was the artificial kidney machine which he had been developing. His strategy was to divest the kidney machine of any mystery at all, for if the Germans had thought it was a secret project it would have been a strong contender for destruction. When shown it, the arrogant German remarked, 'Yes, that is the apparatus I already know from the literature' – which is highly unlikely unless he were the widest read of soldiers. From Kolff's point of view, the man's desire not to reveal his ignorance had the desired effect and the artificial kidney was safe.

Baatz, however, was no fool, and if he kept his silence about any suspicions that the whole inspection might be a charade, it was probably out of a secret respect for Kolff. Baatz later admitted that Sandberg had suspected Kolff was trying to cheat them. Baatz told Kolff, 'I looked him in the face, and just grinned.' Later, Baatz was replaced by Lehrke, and the process of building a working relationship had to begin all over again, made more difficult by Lehrke's resentment of the extra consideration and comparative freedom allowed to doctors.

If Kolff ever came near to arrest and certain deportation to Germany, it was over the escape of two doctors who had been deported from Rotterdam and arrived on Kampen quayside on those infamous barges. With Kolff's help, they had been allowed out of the barracks in order to take a bath at the home of a doctor living in the town. On returning, they walked into the barracks, as they should, but noticed that the Germans guarding the entrance took not the slightest notice of them. Consequently they turned round and walked out again. When their escape was eventually discovered, the Germans ordered that, as compensation, eight senior people from the town should be placed under arrest with a view to being sent with the convoy to Germany. Kolff volunteered himself for arrest. 'I went to the Germans and told them that I knew those two men wanted to escape. "I urged them not to try to escape but they took no notice. But the eight people you have arrested knew nothing about the escape, they are innocent. I knew what they were planning and so if anyone should be arrested, it ought to be me."'

This posed a difficulty for the German commanding officer. 'He was a decent man, and there *were* some decent Germans who weren't true Nazis.' With Kolff he had a working relationship, albeit one based on mutual mistrust. Consequently he was reluctant to have Kolff arrested. Fearing for his own position if it should become known that Kolff had confessed to a part in the doctors' escape, he decided to refer the problem to his senior officers. When they too were unable to make up their minds what to do with Kolff and the eight prisoners, the officer reminded them that Kampen had so far caused little trouble and a random arrest of senior citizens might cause problems where there had been none before. Kolff was off the hook. A long and subtle game with the Nazis, skilfully played out over the miserable years of war, had paid off. Had it not, Kolff would undoubtedly have been arrested and probably shot.

Survival rather than experimentation remained the theme of the last few months of the war. Opportunities to let the inventive mind roam free were rare when so much attention needed to be given to merely staying alive and helping others do the same. No more work was done on the artificial kidney during the remainder of 1944, and it was many months into 1945 before it was wheeled out of the storeroom to be dusted clean of its cobwebs and the rust brushed off. Only then was it found to be heavily damaged: one more victim of the war.

Kolff thought it was time for the wider medical world to read of his experiments, unsuccessful though they had been so far. He penned a preliminary report called, 'The Artificial Kidney'. The final sentence, written in all honesty yet with an underlying optimism, read, 'We must admit that all patients so far treated died. But in so-called hopeless cases we saw some small improvement several times, and we were able to delay death for considerable periods in a number of cases, despite total kidney failure. I do not doubt that sooner or later I shall be able to treat a patient of whom I can say he is cured, and without the artificial kidney he would certainly have died.' He also noted that the tenth patient had, in fact, recovered, but he doubted this was in any way due to his artificial kidney, so he could not claim that as a success. Unaware that these final words would soon have to be rewritten, they were sent to the printer so that Kolff's work could at last become public.

Liberation may have been only a few months away now, but the first four months of 1945 in Holland were worse than any that had gone before. The area around Kampen, being somewhat remote from the main population centres and largely agricultural, may have suffered less than the cities. In Amsterdam, where the daily ration of food was reduced to a hardly sustaining 340 calories, some people were reportedly reduced to eating their family pets. The winter of 1944/5 showed no mercy either, and proved to be desperately cold in a country already perishing through lack of coal and electricity. Schools and factories closed, sewage systems failed in places, rail tracks were vandalised and the sleepers stolen to provide wood for fires. Of the 200,000 Dutch who lost their lives in the Second World War, about 20,000 died during the great 'hunger winter' in a country that was becoming a true hell-hole. Even though the war was turning against them, the Germans did not leave the Netherlands without committing one last act of major destruction. As Canadian troops stormed the north of the country, the Germans systematically destroyed the harbour at Rotterdam and the remaining railway infrastructure. Several dykes were also breached, causing the flooding of thousands of acres of hard-won land.

Kampen's actual moment of liberation, on 17 April 1945, was a muted occasion. Two Canadian army officers rowed sedately across the Ijssel river with the news that the country was once again free. The townspeople gathered to sing 'Abide with Me'. Six weeks later the Kolff family grew again when Kees (short for Cornelius) was born in May 1945. Janke Kolff, who had given birth to five children since 1938 (four of whom survived) must have experienced a gruelling war. She had borne the last three children at eleven-month intervals and had lost her father too. He had joined the resistance at the age of sixty, hoping the Germans would not suspect an older man. His job had been to obtain ration cards for Jews in hiding, but in April 1945, when the war was so nearly over, he was arrested and imprisoned in Apeldoorn. Not long after, when the Allies liberated the town, the prison was found to be empty. Three weeks later the body of Janke's father was found in a mass grave.

Kolff's daughter Adrie reflects that her father '. . . couldn't have done anything without my mother. It wasn't a one-man show. She was there all the time, keeping the show on the road. So vivacious, so full of fun. She wanted to be a wife and a mother more than anything else, and those two things she did to perfection.' Janke Kolff, too, had proved herself a heroine throughout the war years.

8
PEACETIME BRINGS A PATIENT

Kolff must have felt mixed emotions when, in the summer of 1945, with the emotional scars of war still raw, he received news of a possible patient for his artificial kidney, only to discover that the woman was said to have betrayed her own country. Sofia Schafstadt had sympathised with the Germans throughout the long war. Now that the Nazis had been defeated, she had been imprisoned – along with 150,000 others who had shown sympathy to the invaders. Even her own husband had tired of her Nazi sympathies and at one stage during the war had himself locked her up – in the chicken coop.

In Kampen the sympathisers were detained in the town's barracks, recently used to shelter the eight thousand men who had been deported from Rotterdam in the autumn of the previous year. Now the tables had turned and it was a collaborators' prison under the control of Commandant Oudshoorn, a man who had been part of the Dutch underground resistance and was one of the many 'patients' Kolff had helped by inducing false medical symptoms to protect them from deportation to Germany. Oudshoorn decided Schafstadt should be hospitalised as she was clearly a very sick woman.

Dr Kehrer of Kampen Hospital carried out the initial diagnosis on the 67-year-old woman. She was already in a serious condition with a high fever, a distended stomach and a gall bladder so enlarged that it could easily be felt by physical examination. Her skin was yellow and the tiny quantity of urine that she passed was dark brown. Kehrer diagnosed inflammation of the gall bladder, jaundice, kidney failure and uraemia, and commenced treatment with the antibacterial sulphathiazole. (Antibiotics were not yet available.) As Kehrer would have known, it was a characteristic of sulphonamide drugs that they are highly soluble in urine and are rapidly excreted, and so, if Schafstadt was passing no urine because of her kidney failure, the sulphonamide levels in her blood would quickly rise to levels that would do even more damage to her fragile kidneys. For this reason the drug was given for only three days. After eight days she was no better; urine function had not returned and the urea content of her blood was rapidly rising, as were the potassium levels.

Kolff suggested urgent dialysis and asked that the patient be brought to Room 12a, where a newly built artificial kidney had been installed. But Kehrer remained doubtful about the effectiveness of Kolff's invention and persisted with his conventional treatment and even attempted cytoscopy in the hope that it was a mechanical obstruction that was preventing the kidney from working. Kolff could only watch as the condition of the patient worsened. History was repeating itself; the patient was being allowed to deteriorate to a state where nothing on earth could help her. If only he could have the patients *sooner*.

By now Sofia Schafstadt could hardly speak coherently and she slipped in and out of coma. She slept most of the day, snoring very loudly. When the urea level in her blood finally reached a dangerous 4 grams, Kehrer conceded that her kidney function had entirely ceased and that Kolff's machine was now her only hope. This, however, did not represent a new-found faith in Kolff's machine, for he summoned the woman's family to her bedside and addressed them with such finality that they must have gone away with the definite impression that connection to Kolff's kidney machine meant certain death.

Kolff's assistants assembled the artificial kidney for the first time in almost a year; Willy Eskes and Mieneke van der Leij were again put on stand-by in the laboratory with the prospect of long hours ahead of them. The old team fell smoothly into the once-familiar routine. The department of internal medicine's head nurse, Sister M. ter Welle, was there to support Kolff, as she had through so many previous failures. Kolff was to pay tribute to the loyalty of all his staff in the introduction to his thesis. 'My head nurse . . . has been a great support in this work, for the artificial kidney has placed a heavy extra burden on the shoulders of the nurses of the Municipal Hospital of Kampen. I can say that they have all helped enthusiastically; they have kept watch many nights and did not count their fatigue. The two chemical technicians have carried out almost all the determinations mentioned in this thesis. They have always been willing to do chemical analyses whatever the time of day or night.'

The first dialysis lasted for eleven-and-a-half hours, during which Schafstadt developed worrying symptoms. She shook violently, as if chilled, and was warmed with hot water bottles. The blackboard in the kidney room had remained blank for almost a year, but now it started to fill with the cool, clinical details of the levels of urea, potassium and electrolytes in her blood. Kolff watched the all-important urea level and must have wondered if yet another dialysis was doomed to failure. But after nearly eleven hours the patient's blood pressure fell to a more normal level and her blood urea fell to an acceptable 1.2 grams. Kolff disconnected her from the machine and sent her back to a private room. So far, so good. She slept throughout that night and did not stir until the following morning. Kolff was by her bedside at regular intervals and never left the hospital that night.

When she first opened her eyes, it was immediately clear that a dramatic improvement in her condition had occurred. Nevertheless, it was too soon for Kolff to claim any lasting success. The flow of urine was still low and he knew that very soon the toxins would once again start to build up in her bloodstream. He asked for the kidney machine to be prepared for a second dialysis. He worked with determination but great caution: he had been here before and knew how quickly hope could turn to disappointment.

Despite the careful preparation of the cellophane tubing, the mixing of the dialysing fluid and the sterilising of the tubes and connectors, the kidney machine was not switched on again. The patient's own kidneys, without warning, regained their natural function of their own accord and the urine flowed, naturally and unprompted. Sonia Schafstadt was cured, of that there was no doubt: without Kolff's artificial kidney she would undoubtedly have died. Now Kolff had proved what he had set out to establish: that if the sick kidney can be relieved of its work by an artificial organ, then there is a possibility of full recovery in a patient who otherwise would certainly die. He had done it! At last he had avenged the death of young Jan Bruning in Groningen, whose unnecessary demise had inspired Kolff to take the first steps along the long and difficult road that led to the successful dialysis of Sofia Schafstadt that night.

Now it was time to rewrite his thesis, which he had started preparing in the summer of 1945. In the draft that was at that moment being prepared by the printer, Kolff had admitted that so far no life had been saved as a result of his machine. With the confidence inspired by Mrs Schafstadt's treatment, he could now change that concluding paragraph. The printer was urgently contacted and told to hold the last page. Kolff rewrote it to read: 'After the first part of this article was set, such a patient actually came to me . . . the patient was in such desperate condition before treatment with the artificial kidney that we expected her imminent death. With this patient we have in fact provided proof that it is possible to save the life of persons with acute uraemia by use of the artificial kidney . . . she gave us the decisive impetus to continue along the road we had set out on.'

Sofia Schafstadt penned her thoughts too: 'As long as I live I'll never forget my gratitude to Dr Kolff. It's only because of him that I am alive and able to write these lines.' Her medical problems might have been over, but the matter of her freedom was less easily resolved. As a collaborator, she was required to be sent back to the barracks and into the charge of Oudshoorn to await a possible trial for her pro-Nazi activities. Kolff, however, realised that this woman was special; she was the first ever person whose life had been saved by his artificial kidney. He had no wish for her to have uniquely survived kidney failure, only to die in a prison camp through lack of care and attention. Had Kolff been a stranger to Oudshoorn, no doubt Schafstadt would have been taken immediately back to prison, but because of Kolff's help during the war Oudshoorn felt an obligation to the doctor and allowed the woman to go and live with her son in The Hague. She made a rapid recovery and was restored to full health which she enjoyed for a further five years before dying of an illness unrelated to the most celebrated kidney failure in medical history.

However, while it was one thing to achieve his first

successful dialysis, it proved an almost equal task to have it widely accepted for the breakthrough that it was. The long, slow process of persuasion continued in the endless round of meeting doctors, persuading specialists and convincing professors that dialysis was a truly life-saving procedure. Kolff the evangelist briefly took over from Kolff the inventor.

In what proved to be an inspired move, he had already exported four of his kidney machines to locations around the world, for their own safety as much as anything, and these machines were beginning to create interest. One was sent to London's Hammersmith Hospital, where it was under the care of Dr Eric Bywaters, a man who had done much distinguished work on acute renal failure in victims of the London blitz. Bywaters and his team became the third in the world (after Kolff and Alwall) to successfully employ the artificial kidney, as noted in Kolff's 'New Ways of Treating Uraemia', published in 1947. A second machine was sent to Poland but disappeared, only to emerge a few years later in Krakow, where it lay unused owing to lack of funds and expertise. More successful were his placements in the Mount Sinai Hospital in New York and the Royal Victoria Hospital in Montreal.

The installation of the first Canadian kidney machine was greatly helped by the presence of one of Kolff's faithful assistants, Nannie van de Leeuw, who had worked in Kampen alongside Kolff as a student and later as an intern. On arrival in Canada she was given just eleven days in which to get the kidney fully functioning. The success with which she did so is evident from the records of the first three patients to be dialysed. Although the first died, having arrived in the dialysis room in a very poor condition, the second patient recovered fully despite suffering a hefty self-inflicted overdose of a hypnotic drug. Without access to the artificial kidney, he would certainly have died. The third patient, a woman, also arrived in a very poor condition. Her dialysis lasted six hours until her natural kidney function resumed and she left hospital some days later in a good condition. The fourth patient was a young man of twenty who was certainly at death's door, according to his doctors. Nevertheless six hours of dialysis restored his health, and ten days later he was back at work.

Results like these helped to spread the reputation of Kolff's artificial kidney as a true life-saving machine. Soon Kolff's associates were much in demand to share their experience of working not only with the kidney machine but also with its increasingly famous inventor. Kolff recommended that van Noordwijk should head to Toronto to join a research team working on dialysis techniques using heparin and cellophane. Here, van Noordwijk was to build an artificial kidney from scratch, all the models donated by Kolff having been put to use elsewhere.

In Kampen Kolff's restless mind had moved on. He wanted to know, in the new post-war atmosphere, how information could once again be freely exchanged, and whether others had also been working on an artificial kidney, and if so with what success. He turned to a British information service in Holland which scanned the medical journals for articles that might suggest others had been pursuing similar lines of research to his own. They came up with nothing. In fact, others *had* been working on very similar lines, notably Nils Alwall, in Sweden, who had been constructing artificial kidneys since 1942, but employing them only in the treatment of animals until he was satisfied they were safe for human use. He didn't publish his paper until 1947, and was followed in 1948 by Murray in Toronto who was working on similar lines. If it were a horse-race to determine who invented the world's first artificial kidney, doubtless it would have ended in a photofinish. Who can be certain which papers would have hit the printing press first had not all this research been conducted under the restrictions of world war?

In the event, the honour goes to Kolff.

9
NIGHT TRAINS AND NEW IDEAS

Kolff sensed that he now had the ammunition to win the battle for acceptance of his machine world-wide. His thesis had been well received after deep and critical analysis and he was awarded his doctorate in medicine 'cum laude'. One question remained: here was a young and ambitious doctor at the height of his inventive powers. His creation of the artificial kidney bore the hallmarks not of the summit to a career, but rather of a promising beginning. What was he going to do next?

Life in Holland was slowly improving after the ravages of war and was returning to some kind of normality. Kolff sent his eldest son Jack for carpentry lessons from a wagon builder, hoping perhaps that the love of working with wood might pass from father to son. The cold, snowy winters made for good skating along the canals, and the annual traditional hunt for the first *kiewiet* (lapwing) eggs of the season, suspended during the war, resumed. It was a tradition that the first egg found was presented to the Queen of the Netherlands; tradition also demanded that when the egg was discovered, usually by a farmer, it was carried carefully rolled in the brim of his cap and taken safely home. Kolff's daughter Adrie remembers that for children the hardest part of the egg hunt was the crossing of the ditches and canals, which they achieved with the help of stout poles stabbed deep into the bed of the canal by the adults. Catapult-like, the pole was pulled back, the child held on, and when the pole was released the child was hopefully propelled across to the far bank. 'The tricky part was clinging on. It was slippery and well polished with use and not made for a child's hand.'

Family life was soon to be suspended, though, for both parents were to disappear from their children's lives. Kolff's scientific papers were beginning to arouse great interest in the USA, and an invitation from fellow Dutchman Isador Snapper, Professor of Medicine at Mount Sinai Hospital, led to a major tour of the States in March 1947 during which Kolff could not only lecture on his work but also instruct others in the use of his artificial kidney. Snapper saw great virtue in the way the Americans organised their medical research, with much to commend in the way medical schools were closely associated with private universities, and was impressed that industrial sponsorship of medical research was not shunned. He liked the way that teachers of medicine could work full time at education and not have to manage a private practice to earn a wage. During the war Snapper had been captured by the Japanese and was exchanged by the Dutch for a captured Japanese general. Freed by his captors, Snapper went to the USA as a consultant to the surgeon-general of the army and became director of medical education at the Mount Sinai Hospital, to which Kolff had sent one of his early artificial kidneys. Snapper was brilliant, if arrogant. One of his students remembers asking, 'How can it be that you are not certified by the American Board of Internal Medicine?', to which the reply from Snapper was, 'Who on the board would dare to examine me?'

Kolff doubtless fell under Snapper's spell. His charisma was never in question. His belief that modern diagnostic methods were much devalued if they were not employed alongside Hippocratic empirical medicine – in other words, the bedside manner still had much to commend it in a rapidly advancing medical age – was Kolff's belief too. Kolff remembers: 'I offered Snapper an artificial kidney which I had made, and I very much wanted to go to New York to show them how to use it. Snapper said he would pay for my stay in New York, so off it went and when I arrived the kidney was waiting for me. I remember it was the model with wooden laths because we couldn't get hold of aluminium then. Snapper and I had much in common, he greeted me with great warmth. As my sponsor, he was much concerned that I make the best possible impression upon his colleagues. He asked to see the lecture I was going to give and he was horrified that I was going to deliver it off the cuff, as my old teacher Brinkman had taught me. He insisted I sat down right there and then, in the hotel room, and write out the lecture for him. I obliged, although I have always wondered why he was so apprehensive about my powers. I guessed it must be because I came from Kampen – a place that was legendary for its fools!'

The lecture proved a huge success and was the start of a theatrical series of appearances by Kolff, whose reputation was spreading. With his wife Janke, he was away from the Netherlands for three months in 1947, shifting from hotel to hotel, managing on very little money to cover their travelling costs, delivering the lecture, then catching the night train to be ready for the next appearance. 'In Boston,' Kolff remembers, 'I was the guest of Dr George Thorn at the Peter Bent Brigham Hospital, but I was unable to offer them an artificial kidney because I had already given them all away. So I gave a set of plans to a young doctor called Joseph Murray who was anxious to experiment with artificial kidneys. Together with one of the surgeons there, Carl Walter, he made modifications and this version became known as the Kolff/Brigham Artificial Kidney.' In fact, the redesign led to major improvements, and several dozen were built and sent all over the world.

The principal legacies of Kolff's visit were the first successful dialysis carried out in the USA at the Mount Sinai Hospital in New York in 1948, and the launching of Murray on an outstanding career as a nephrologist. Later, in 1954, Murray was to perform the first successful kidney transplantation between identical twins at the Peter Bent Brigham Hospital in Boston, for which he was awarded the Nobel Prize.

It was also in 1948 that Kolff was given the Amory Award in Boston, together with Waksam (who had developed the antibiotic streptomycin) and Papanicolaou (who devised the cervical smear). Kolff was now recognised as a true innovator.

One other defining event happened on that tour of the USA, and it happened on the night train from Chicago to Minneapolis. Kolff remembers waking in the night, as he did so often when inspiration was about to strike. Turning to Janke he said, 'I have thoughts of building an oxygenator.' In his hand was a length of crinkled sausage skin, which again was to be the basis of his new machine. Janke groaned, knowing only too well what life was like with an inventive man grasping at a new idea. Kolff remembers her saying only, 'Oh God, not again!' before her head slumped back on the pillow in despair.

Kolff's oxygenator, a device on which others around the world had already done some pioneering work, was to be his *second* artificial organ. It took shape in the sort of makeshift conditions which he had to endure for much of his working life. His laboratory at Kampen Hospital was sandwiched halfway between the morgue and the garage, with a connecting window between. Jack Kolff, then aged eight, remembers, 'My father used to take me on the back of his bike to see his office and then sometimes we would go down to his laboratory. I saw all the experiments he was doing. I remember once seeing lots of blood and lots of foam. I didn't know it then, but I guess now that he was working on some kind of oxygenator.'

During the very first dialysis Kolff had noticed that the blood which had been taken from a vein became more vivid in colour as it passed through the artificial kidney, and by the time it emerged at the far end of the cellophane tubing it had the appearance of arterial blood – it had been oxygenated. Could it be that he had coincidentally invented the artificial lung? That thought first occurred to him when he noticed that change in colour of the blood, and he stored away that nugget and held on to it until after his tenth attempt at dialysis, after which he turned to Bob van Noordwijk and whispered, 'Now I know how to make the connections for my artificial heart.' It was a throwaway remark, but it laid the foundations for the rest of his working life.

The invention of the artificial heart had effectively begun even before Kolff's artificial kidney had been perfected. As Jack Kolff, now a heart surgeon, observes of his father, 'He recognised that the kidney, heart and lungs are all related. If you're using a pump to push blood through an artificial kidney, what's the difference between that and an artificial heart? You're handling it, moving it, oxygenating it, warming it, cooling it. All part of the same problem, and he saw that. That understanding of the simple but fundamental association between the functioning of those organs is what made him a great inventor.' Or as Kolff himself explained it to me, rather more dryly, 'How does the body know where the blood is coming from?'

The juxtaposition of his laboratory and the hospital's morgue provided Kolff with a unique, if macabre, opportunity. Kolff had often remarked that in Kampen he had an unprecedented freedom to carry out his experiments. He had neither to justify nor explain, only to do what he thought was best for his patients. He alone decided what was right and wrong. In more modern times a medical authority might view with scepticism some of his experiments, but then, as Kolff remarks, 'Nobody tried to stop me doing anything.'

His experiments involved the insertion of canulas into the veins and arteries of cadavers in order to assess the correct sizes to use, and the ideal places to use them. At that time family consent did not seem to enter into it and so these experiments were not without their grim excitement. Once, while taking the opportunity to investigate a body that was lying in the mortuary awaiting its funeral, he heard the sound of horses' hooves echoing along the cobbled Kampen streets that led round the back of the hospital. It was the turn of his own blood to freeze in his veins. He hardly dared breathe. Through the closed and bolted mortuary door, he heard the family announce that they had come to view the body of their loved one. 'We were struck with terror', remembers Kolff. But the staff of the hospital were immensely loyal, and the family was told that only the head nurse held the key to the morgue and she had gone shopping. The family said they would return later that day. Kolff breathed again.

The oxygenation of blood now excited him, and he believed that by combining such a device with a pump he could take the very first steps towards an artificial heart/lung machine. His object now was to show that he could oxygenate 5 litres of blood per minute. Others, notably the Swedish scientist Viking Olov Bjork, had tried this before, and the result had been the disc oxygenator which consisted of twenty revolving plates on an axle sitting in a bath of blood. As the discs rotated, a thin film of blood attached itself to them, and as the blood-covered discs emerged into the oxygen-filled chambers oxygenation took place. It was, according to Kolff, a good machine but it did enormous physical damage to the blood proteins. In his endless quest for cheaper medicine, he built a version of that oxygenator employing discarded Dictaphone discs instead of expensive and scarce stainless steel.

Kolff's quest was now for a more benign device which could oxygenate the blood while causing the minimum of physical damage. He believed that cellophane membranes again held the key. However, unlike his artificial kidney, human experiment was out of the question. Instead, a deal was struck with the Food Rationing Bureau, which arranged for a fifth cow to be added to the city's weekly ration of four cows for slaughter. On this fifth cow Kolff was to conduct his experiment, with the slaughterman standing by so that should the cow show the slightest sign of distress it could be immediately dispatched.

In typical Kolff fashion, the prototype oxygenator which he wished to test had been constructed with the aid of much lateral thinking. On a visit to Sweden to visit Bjork, Kolff was impressed with the notion of applying the action of an agricultural milking machine to the problem of moving blood through the body if the heart were bypassed. On returning home, he obtained such a machine from Alfa Laval in nearby Zwolle, and set about making modifications. Why not reverse the milking machine, he thought, to make it pump rather than suck, and so replicate the action of the heart? This he did, and in the subsequent experiment conducted on the cow he proved that when the animal was deprived of oxygen from its own lungs, its blood could receive enough oxygen via his machine to keep it alive for no less than fifteen minutes. After the experiment, 'it was killed and eaten'. It did not die in vain, for a whole new era of cardiac surgery was about to be opened up, in which it had played a modest but vital part.

Filled with enthusiasm at the prospect of a second artificial organ, Kolff gave a lecture to the University of Leiden entitled 'Life Without Heart and Kidneys'. But no matter how much the pursuit of artificial organs excited him, there was little prospect of further research in an impoverished post-war country. Moreover, Kolff's achievements were not fully appreciated by all of his peers. One of the Netherlands' most prominent kidney specialists, Professor Borst, a survivor of wartime imprisonment, apparently remained unconvinced even by Kolff's successful treatment of Sofia Schafstadt, and said so publicly. At a medical conference in Utrecht where Kolff preached the virtues of his machine, Borst was quick to quash his enthusiasm. In retaliation, Kolff stood up and declared, with his tongue firmly in his cheek, 'Like all Dutchmen I rejoice that Professor Borst has been freed from the concentration camp. That was a great day for Dutch medicine. But as far as the artificial kidney is concerned, he might have stayed there a while longer.' The audience laughed and Borst too was quick to see the joke. In fact, his opinion mellowed and he admitted that the kidney machine might, after all, have virtue.

There were other signs too that it was time for Kolff to move on. 'I feared that the Russians would come', he remembers. 'A lot of people at the time were of the same mind. There were Roman Catholic priests who'd prayed for Hitler to win the war because he was better than the Russians. I also thought that having lost its colonies, Holland was doomed to poverty for the foreseeable future. So, when I see a possibility to do something worthwhile, I have to do it.'

Doubtless flattered by the attention he had received in the USA, and enjoying the almost celebrity status he now held, for Kolff it seemed that crossing the Atlantic with his wife and children was the right thing to do. But in Kampen he had been king, an almost God-like figure in the town's hospital who had been allowed, sometimes under sufferance, to pursue his researches and his ostensibly mad ideas. In America he was to find himself not at the top of the ladder, but back on the very bottom rung once again. Nevertheless, the words of Professor Snapper repeated themselves in his head: 'Even if you only find a chair to sit on, you should come to America.'

The two eldest children, Jack and Adrie, who were grown up enough to understand what it meant to move to America, were thrilled by the idea. A fifth child, Therus, had been born in Holland in June 1949, and all five children stayed at home with their mother while Kolff headed westwards. In Kampen, Janke was left to cope with the five youngsters, and to come to terms with the impending upheaval in their lives, although there was now no money in the bank to fund the move. Kolff had been in America for two weeks when he called to say the two eldest children, Jack and Adrie, should be sent straight away. He had found families with whom they could stay, and life for them 'would be better'. Janke did not relish the idea of dispatching two children 'like orphans on a 17-hour journey by propeller-driven plane'. 'We went to America', remembers Adrie, 'with little bags on strings round our necks with our money in them.' Jack, then eleven, had an ambition to 'help support the family by raising chickens'.

Kolff himself had been unable to secure a position in a university because of the large numbers of American servicemen returning from Korea who had been promised a full education in return for their efforts. As a result, there were few academic places for immigrants. Kolff, however, was happy to find a place at the Cleveland Clinic in Ohio, a centre of medical excellence where the research department was under the charge of Irvine Page, an already distinguished figure whose speciality was hypertension. Kolff reasoned that the marriage of his work on the artificial kidney with Page's expertise in high blood pressure would enable them to co-operate in establishing a centre of world excellence. That remained to be seen.

From young Jack Kolff's point of view, there was nowhere better to be than in America. He and his sister Adrie, now ten, had long been on the receiving end of relief parcels sent after the war. 'It was like Christmas every time we opened one', remembers Jack, who was convinced that all good things in the world came from America. This was entirely due to the efforts of their Aunt Mimi, the daughter of Cornelius G. Kolff (after whom one of the Staten Island ferries was named). He had founded the Staten Island Chamber of Commerce and was responsible in the late nineteenth century for thirty-six residential developments which fuelled a property boom that lasted well into the 1920s. As a wheeler-dealer in land and property, there were few developers in Staten Island more astute than Kolff. 'Aunt Mimi was *very high* Kolff', Jack remembers. 'She even had escutcheons on the dinner plates. That's how seriously she took being a Kolff!' She never married and would have been the last of the American Kolffs had not a new contingent arrived from Holland to continue the family line. This may have been part of the reason for her generous welcome.

For the children it was 'exciting to be in America, but confusing and disorientating. I suddenly became no more than a little immigrant', remembers Adrie. 'Although I didn't know it at the time, it set both of us back years in terms of our self-confidence.' Adrie went to live with the family occupying the house that was later to become the Kolff family home; Jack went to live with a family where there were more boys to keep him company. Six weeks after their arrival, when the house was ready, Janke and the three remaining boys joined them after a gruelling flight and overnight train journey, Janke struggling to cope with her tired and fractious youngest in the blazing heat of a June day. It must have seemed considerably less of an adventure for her.

Kolff's salary was not huge – only $8,000 a year, which was less than he had earned in Kampen – and barely enough to support a family of seven. Janke's inheritance seems to have been spent by now, and a loan from one of Kolff's brothers had helped to pay for the house. Nevertheless, Janke was expected to keep up the domestic standards which Kolff had enjoyed in the Netherlands. She soon realised that, unlike back home, they could afford no servant to help. Tough days lay ahead.

They lived in an old colonial-style house, built of wood, three storeys high, and backed by tall elm trees. Alas, the paint was peeling and there was no money to pay for a decorator. Janke soon found herself up a ladder, brush in hand, taking advice from a bemused neighbour who gently advised her that you have to remove the old paint first! Janke remembers this as an endless operation and didn't take kindly to Kolff's contribution, which was the present of an electric paint remover for her birthday. It was, indeed, a very different life for all of them, and especially for the Dutch-born children, for whom the perplexing process of comprehending baseball was just beginning.

10

THE KING OF KAMPEN
LOSES HIS CROWN

Kolff, freshly arrived from the Netherlands, soon found
that the welcome Aunt Mimi had laid on for his children
was not matched by his reception at the Cleveland Clinic.
For the first two years he was 'very depressed'. Yet no
matter how great a struggle life might become, he knew
that there was no possibility of ever going back to Europe.
'I never thought for one moment that I'd made the wrong
choice.' In moments of doubt, Snapper was quick to
remind him that some academics in the Netherlands did
not fully appreciate Kolff's practical approach, preferring a
purer, more clinical attitude. 'I wasn't considered scientific
enough for Holland. I was seen as being focused on
practical solutions to clinical problems.' It was a view not
widely shared among the medical establishment in the
Netherlands, but undoubtedly there were some who
thought Kolff was obsessed with *gadgets*. Kolff is quick to
point out that they failed to realise that it was *gadgets* that
opened up whole new fields in medicine and that
biochemistry only moved forward after someone invented
a gadget able to determine carbon dioxide.

As his son Jack observes, 'In Kampen he could do what
he liked, but when he got to Cleveland he was little more
than a resident with a research lab. For a start he had to
learn to do his own typing. I remember he even took a
typewriter on holiday with him. It was painful to watch. Of

course, he didn't have a licence to practice medicine in the USA and so he had to go back to the text books and pass the exams.'

There was more disappointment in store. The head of research, the distinguished Irvine Page, whom Kolff remembers as a good-looking man with the talent to be a jazz singer, proved to be more distant professionally than Kolff had expected. 'I'd told him that with our combined specialities of kidney dialysis and hypertension, we could make a great team. But he didn't seem interested.' The research department was a good one, and many residents came to work there for little pay, but it was soon noticed that when Kolff was doing hospital rounds, five or six researchers would attach themselves to him, while some of the less charismatic but senior doctors were left with none. 'I don't think I was popular in the research department. It was the time of the Korean War and they wanted to use my rotating drum kidney in the field. But when they chose someone to send out there to advise, I was overlooked. It was very painful. It was seven years before they even let me have a secretary.'

Kolff thought he would be welcomed at Cleveland, but clearly there was going to be no red carpet laid out for him. But Kolff persisted, as was his way, and when the wife of the colorectal surgeon, Rupert Turnbull, became seriously ill, it was a chance for Kolff to make a reputation for himself. 'She had haemorrhaged in childbirth,' he remembers, 'and the chief of the department of surgery said to me, "See that she's treated properly".' After Kolff's repeated trips to the distant hospital in which she was a patient, the surgeon's wife made a good recovery, largely thanks to his detailed attention, and word soon spread through the Cleveland Clinic that this immigrant was to be trusted.

His new-found reputation did little to improve his working conditions which, compared with Kampen, verged on the unworkable. Having little sympathy with Kolff's artificial kidneys, Page was disinclined to provide him with much working space. 'When I came to Cleveland, I was given a laboratory on the sixth floor, which I had to share with a physicist called Olmsted, a man who became a great help to me. He had one half of the room, I had the other. The clinic had a version of my artificial kidney made by Allis-Chalmers, and I equipped my half of the laboratory so that patients could be dialysed there.'

This proved to be a far from easy process, for not only was it the most inconvenient treatment room in the entire hospital, but it also housed other procedures besides Kolff's artificial kidney experiments. His main aim in coming to Cleveland in the first place was to develop his heart/lung machine, working eventually towards an artificial heart. In developing both these devices he carried out his experiments on dogs. These too had to share the kidney room with the human patients, while the long-suffering physicist fitted in as best he could. 'To get a patient into that laboratory so they could be treated with the artificial kidney, we had to carry them from the north wing of the hospital, through a narrow corridor, down four steps, then around a tight corner and finally into the room. Of course, when a patient came to us we had to get rid of the dogs and make the place sterile, clean the laboratory, disassemble the bed for transport, reassemble it in the laboratory, carry the patient in, dialyse the patient and then carry them all the way back. Also, while we were treating the patients, the experiments on the dogs came to a halt and we lost valuable data and much had to be repeated.'

Eventually Kolff was given a laboratory more conveniently placed on the second floor, but this too was hardly ideal and underlined how little value was placed on his work. He was obliged to share this new room with a neurosurgeon called W. James Gardner, whose theory of a novel treatment for burns victims was to prove somewhat intrusive. 'His idea was to suspend them in a fluid in which they would be practically weightless, and to do that he had a tank made in which the patient could be held vertically with only their head visible. The fluid in which they floated consisted of an oil bath, and the theory was that urine and other body waste would sink to the bottom of the tank while the oil above would remain relatively clean.' To test his theory – and this is where it verges on high farce – new surgical residents were invited to spend twenty-four hours in the tank so as to fully understand the sensation and be able to describe it to prospective patients. In the end the treatment didn't work, but it caused Kolff no small inconvenience while in development – not least the haunting looks that must have shadowed the faces of the volunteer residents as they counted the minutes until they were free from this oily torture.

To further emphasise Kolff's diminished status at the Cleveland Clinic, he remembers that when Irvine Page went to visit his own research department, he used to walk down the corridor that passed Kolff's laboratory. 'Often there were one or two artificial kidneys in the hallway, and I remember the mere sight of them irritated Page beyond belief. He always went out of his way to shove, push and kick them aside.' The King of Kampen had truly lost his crown.

His time was not wasted, though. In fact, despite the pressures of adjusting to an alien working atmosphere, it was an extraordinarily productive period for Kolff. He never forgot that his main aim in coming to the USA was to perfect his heart/lung machine. Like others engaged in similar research around the world, he believed that a whole new era of surgery would be introduced if it were possible for surgeons to replicate the function of the heart using a machine, while at the same time stopping the natural heart and surgically repairing it. He had shown with his kidney machine that the patient's blood was dark red (oxygen-poor) when it entered the cellophane tubing of his artificial kidney, but had turned bright red (oxygen-rich) by the time it emerged at the far end. In Kampen his experiments on the cow had shown that by the use of pumps he could oxygenate 5 litres per minute, which was sufficient to give his machine a clinical application. But there was much work to do in perfecting the pumps to prevent physical damage to the blood, and in the design and operation of the crude oxygenators he had brought over from Kampen.

However, a new surgical technique developed by Dr Charles Bailey, working in Philadelphia in 1948, briefly cast doubt over whether a heart/lung machine would ever be needed. Bailey had devised a technique for working inside the heart without first having to stop it: the technique was called mitral commissurotomy, and was used in the first ever successful attempt at surgery on heart valves. According to Kolff, 'Bailey's technique involved putting two gloves over the surgeon's hand. The tip of the index finger was cut off the outer glove and a knife blade was shoved between the two layers. After finding the mitral valve, which he reached through the atrium, he then advanced the blade of the knife so that the tip of it emerged between the inner and outer rubber glove. Then he could cut the commissure, the tissue which was preventing the proper functioning of the valve.'

This sounded all very well on paper, but Bailey's technique was controversial and mortality rates were high. Because of his repeated lack of success he was about to lose his privileges, so Bailey arranged for three patients to be operated on in rapid succession in three different hospitals, employing the tried and tested principle that a moving target was harder to hit. He performed the first operation and the patient died. The second patient died too. But before he could be prevented from performing a third operation, the unstoppable Charles Bailey was proceeding with all haste to the Episcopal Hospital in Philadelphia, where his third patient was waiting for him. As he stood over the operating table with his double gloved hand hovering above his patient, a representative of the hospital authority burst into the operating room and announced, 'Dr Bailey, you cannot do that!' to which he replied, 'I just have.' The patient survived, and so proud was Bailey that only one week after the operation, he took the patient to Chicago to parade him before the American Medical Association Convention. The fact that Dr Dwight Harken of Boston, who performed a similar operation only six days later, was also appearing at the convention may have inspired Bailey to remind his distinguished audience that he was the real pioneer of the technique, if only by a week.

Proper open heart surgery, where the heart is drained of blood and stopped, required more than just a new surgical technique. It needed a machine to carry out the workload of the heart for the duration of the operation. Kolff was not the first in this field of heart/lung machine development, although he could justifiably claim to have been the first to recognise the oxygenating potential of his early artificial kidney. In 1953, during Kolff's early years at Cleveland, Dr John Gibbon had employed a heart/lung machine for the first time ever in open-heart surgery, and he is the true pioneer. His device was a screen oxygenator in which a thin film of blood cascaded down a metal screen surrounded by oxygen. It was a temperamental device, by all accounts, and it was difficult to guarantee an even spread of the blood across the screen. Kolff remembers it as 'a superb machine, if complicated'.

Gibbon's first open-heart operation using a heart/lung machine was on an eighteen-year-old girl with right-side heart failure. The defect was corrected in forty-five minutes and the girl made a full recovery. Unlike many competitive medical researchers and inventors in America at the time, Gibbon was described as being 'modest to a fault'. The leading cardiac surgeon, Denton Cooley, who was later to become an artificial heart pioneer, said of him, 'He led a life without any need whatsoever of being the slightest bit conniving in order to make a good mark on the world, to be accepted, to gain approval.' He describes him as 'a surgeon who wanted to be a poet'. After performing the world's first bypass-assisted open-heart operation, he only 'let a few friends know about the operation. That was all.' A truly modest surgeon. With his second patient, however, he was not as successful, and the patient died. Gibbon took the loss badly, and didn't give the oxygenator so much as a second glance for a whole year.

If Kolff lagged behind him in his researches, it was not by many months, and the first use of a Kolff membrane oxygenator happened almost by accident. The major problem with his membrane-based designs remained the difficulty of oxygenating sufficient blood to keep a fully grown patient alive. In experiments on dogs Kolff had shown that in a creature with a small circulation his machine had the efficiency required. He had been conducting an experiment in which he replaced the cellophane membrane in his oxygenator with polyethylene (thus forsaking sausage skin forever) and had called in a colleague to come and observe the progress of a dog on the operating table. The animal was connected to

Kolff's oxygenator and its heart was being operated upon, but Dr Soames saw more than merely the animal before him, and declared, 'This is it!'

He had realised that although the machine lacked the capacity to oxygenate an adult human, it would certainly be sufficient for an infant. With Kolff's apparatus, he might be able to operate on a very young child which had been born with a congenital heart defect and required immediate surgery.

Kolff was unsure, and reluctant to allow his machine to be tested on something as fragile as a baby while he still considered it to be in the early stages of development. Soames consulted the chief of cardiovascular surgery, Dr Effler, and convinced him that an operation *was* possible using this machine. Effler agreed and said he would do the operation himself. Kolff remained unpersuaded that his machine was ready for a human trial, and struck a deal: if he could perform an open-heart procedure on ten dogs and they all survived, he would allow his machine to be used on a child.

Ten dogs were prepared. The operations were done in rapid succession. First they were put on the oxygenator, then the chest was opened. The heart was opened and then sewn up again to replicate an open-heart operation, and the chest was then closed. To Kolff's great satisfaction all ten dogs survived. He describes with enormous pleasure a home movie taken of the ten young dogs, crammed in a basket, biting the others' ears, playing and cavorting like healthy young dogs do. He now felt able to give his approval to the first use of his membrane oxygenator on a human patient.

Sadly, the baby on which the first operation was performed died – but the second and third survived, and both lived healthy lives thereafter. This would not have been possible without Kolff's oxygenator. Yet again, a device of Kolff's invention, an artificial organ operating outside the body, had saved human life.

Inspired, he now started to develop larger machines, based on the ones first devised in Kampen in which he had proved that he could oxygenate the required volume of blood to maintain the circulation of a cow – or a fully grown person. These machines were gathering dust in the basement of the Cleveland Clinic, the surgeons preferring the 'blind' techniques developed by Bailey. 'Why use Kolff's damned machines when we can do it so simply?' they argued. But it soon became clear that blind surgery techniques had their limits, and perhaps Kolff's oxygenators had their uses after all.

The pressure under which technicians were required to work in bringing Kolff's machines into practical use shouldn't be underestimated. These were new techniques requiring the utmost vigilance. Kolff remembers that for the early open-heart operations, there were no fewer than sixteen people involved. It was the technicians' job to prepare the oxygenator and prime it with blood so that both machine and patient were ready for the surgeon on his arrival. He remembers a precise protocol being established: 'One of the rules was that if the surgeon, who was of course in total command of the surgery, said something, the person to whom it was addressed had to repeat it to make sure he'd heard it and understood it. I wrote out a list of commandments and hung them near the overhead light in the operating room. They read: "Repeat the order of the surgeon. No irrelevant talk. Be alert for the mistakes of others and be ready to speak about it."'

There are never any guarantees with novel procedures conducted with groundbreaking equipment, and failure was inevitable. The membrane oxygenators which Kolff had developed, and which had been successfully used on children, were proving too small for use on adults; sufficient capacity could be achieved by stacking several machines together, but this was too bulky. To solve the problem of building larger oxygenators, Kolff characteristically looked outside the medical establishment, and this time he turned to heavy industry. He secured the services of the 'marvellous and gifted' engineer Larry Hursic, from the Acme Company in Cleveland, whose last job had been the engineering of the immense shears used to cut metal waste into manageable chunks prior to melting – they were principally used in the car crushing business. The parallels between such heavy engineering and the more delicate management of human blood might have escaped most people, but Kolff recognised a novel talent when he saw it and the Acme engineer duly joined his team. His specific task was to build roller pumps, which were more efficient than the air-driven pumps of the milking machines which had been used until now in the smaller, membrane oxygenators. As Kolff remarked, 'He built it according to my wishes and my dreams.' The major problem proved to be the volume of blood required to prime it. Filling the machine without introducing bubbles was also a difficulty that had to be resolved, otherwise the blood returning to the patient would be lethal. Kolff reasoned that if the machine could be reversed while being set up, and the blood was sucked back into the machine rather than pumped through it, then the bubble problem would be reduced. A simple reversing switch would achieve this.

The first patient was made ready for surgery, and a technician prepared the machine and attached the patient. No one guessed there was any problem. But on opening the heart, the surgeon complained that there was too much blood for him to operate and that somehow the blood was not being removed. They guessed the pump was underpowered and that the machine needed to run faster, so the speed of the pumps was increased. The situation only became worse. 'By now the surgeon was screaming bloody murder, which it was', admits Kolff. What was happening, he later found out, was that the blood was being pumped back into the patient instead of out. The switch on the machine had been left in reverse. The instant the problem was detected the switch was thrown, but the damage had already been done and the blood in the pulmonary veins had backed up into the venous system of the lungs and destroyed the capillaries. 'That evening, at ten o'clock,' Kolff remembers, 'the patient, a young boy, said to me, "I can breathe but I cannot get the oxygen out." The boy died and I still feel terrible about it. But if you start new procedures, you run some risks. I made a very simple change in the machine and that was to put a large red handle over the switch and you could not reverse the machine without the operator holding that handle. But for that poor boy it was too late.'

Other problems presented themselves. It was found that in early open-heart operations, when the heart had been stopped, unintentional damage could be done to a collection of heart muscle fibres, known as the Bundle of His. These fibres carried the 'messages' from the atria to the ventricles without which the heart could not beat properly. But because the heart had been stopped by the surgeon to carry out his operation, any unintentional damage to the messenger nerves was not recognised until attempts were made to restart the heart, which would prove difficult for reasons that would not be apparent. Kolff decided a pacemaker would solve the problem in such patients, and applied to Page to be allowed to employ one if necessary. Page, the head of research, said that since the pacemaker was not part of a research programme, he wasn't going to pay for it. Never able to accept defeat after the first round of a fight, Kolff went straight to the head of medicine, who also declined Kolff's request on the basis of his belief that there is no fault in the beating of the heart which cannot be cured with medicine, *not* with machines. Kolff, convinced that a pacemaker was required, turned to the physicist Rick Olmsted, with whom he had shared the laboratory, and asked him to build one. The result was hardly a compact device, but it was an effective one, despite having long leads which emerged from the patient's chest, travelled out of the operating room, along the corridors and eventually to the recovery room where the controls were set up. Kolff says that they later refined it to the point where the device was small enough to implant into a child. However, despite its clear commercial value, Kolff never took out a patent nor sought commercial gain. The same was true of his dialysers and oxygenators. The making of money from medical inventions was never high on his agenda and the Cleveland Clinic did not allow it. Nor did it permit patent applications, believing that medical research was performed for the free benefit of all mankind. Kolff agreed with this.

It is difficult to imagine Kolff involved in any form of relaxation, or to believe that the inventive inclination of his mind ever took time off. But he was a father of five, and family life had to be maintained, although his duties at the Cleveland Clinic gave little scope for family recreation. At Janke's insistence he avoided the round of weekend cocktail parties which were a pastime of the medical community. Instead, he played with his children. 'There was never to be any medical talk in front of the children,' remembers Janke, 'no child can grow in the shade of an enormous tree.'

These were often stressful times, and the dutiful Janke was Kolff's strength and support, cooking supper at short notice for various research colleagues, being at home for the children, attending to the kitchen sink duties – which Kolff shunned. 'Sometimes,' she says, 'I was so tired that I just lay down flat on the floor. I survived on willpower and physical strength and music.'

Kolff and Janke thought life might be better spent partially outside Cleveland itself, and while the rest of his family were away in Holland in 1958 (their first visit since emigrating), Kolff made a search of north-east Ohio, looking for land. He found 92 acres on the Grand River, complete with a ramshackle farmhouse, a deep ravine and a creek. 'I sent a telegram to Janke, in the Netherlands, asking permission to buy the land with money she had inherited. I didn't have the money, she did. I got permission, with love, and the land was ours.'

Then followed an urgent restoration. 'I was in deadly fear that my wife Janke and the children would come back from the Netherlands before the farmhouse was painted. It hadn't seen any paint for forty years and was in terrible shape. So I invited all the fellows of the Cleveland Clinic to come over at weekends. One or two were assigned to cook hamburgers and the others were given large cans with white paint and brushes and were invited to paint. Foreign medical doctors hadn't been trained in painting or to stand on ladders, but they learnt! I found one little Japanese doctor on top of a very high ladder which was standing on a large round stone – two other Japanese tried to keep the legs in place to stop him falling over. The farm was a joy for everybody. I remember Dr Akutsu; he was able to split a log, holding the wood with one foot so the axe would pass about two inches ahead from his toes!'

The farm was to become something of a weekend haven. Adrie remembers loving the place. 'It was an L-shaped house, with a porch, and in Prohibition days it had been a distillery – we found empty bottles. Dad and mother threw themselves into the place, buying a tractor and a mower, building a pond and stocking it with fish. My mother used to cook good, fast meals for us. Great days.'

Although on Janke's insistence medical talk was forbidden, some of Kolff's fellow researchers, who were also family friends, came to stay. Some visitors, however, remember these supposedly relaxing weekends as being something of a trial, believing that surviving the weekend was as much a part of Kolff's assessment of them as a medical exam might be. One recalled, 'I was invited to the farm as a prospective colleague and I thought I would be talking medicine with him and discussing ideas and prospective projects. But all I seemed to do the whole weekend was stir a big pot of pea soup. But I had the feeling he was watching the way I stirred it, trying to arrive at some judgement about how I used my hands, perhaps.'

If an atmosphere of willing co-operation, which he had enjoyed and been stimulated by in Kampen, eluded him in Cleveland, his capacity for invention was in no way stifled. In 1955, when you might think his work on the heart/lung machine would give him no time for anything else, he came up with a totally new idea – a disposable artificial kidney. It was a joint invention with Dr Bruno Watschinger, an Austrian who had come to Cleveland to research hypertension in the context of renal failure, and in particular to work alongside Page, who was considered a world authority on the subject. Watschinger knew about Kolff's rotating kidney – indeed, Kolff had encouraged him to use it – but such an apparatus was far too expensive for post-war Austria to consider. When he voiced these reservations, Kolff's reaction was, 'So then, let us make one which is cheap to build!'

An economical, possibly disposable, kidney satisfied in Kolff the desire to perfect even further his own invention, and to ensure that it should be available as widely and as cheaply to as many patients as possible. Cheap, easily available treatment had always been one of Kolff's pursuits, and in the disposable kidney he thought he had found it. Typically Page was less than impressed. When Kolff asked for time to work on it, Page gave him three weeks. Watschinger, on a three-month stipend funded by the World Health Organisation, became his collaborator.

The idea was to use materials of the utmost simplicity. In 1953 another artificial kidney had been invented by Inouye and Engelberg. They wound cellulose tubing around a core and immersed it in a pressure cooker. This simple idea had great Kolff appeal. One lunchtime, while Kolff and Watschinger were discussing what to use for a core, their eyes fell upon an empty pineapple juice can. This became the basis of the twin-coil kidney – simply because two coils of cellulose tubing were wound round the juice can.

His children were unfailing in their support and were happy to empty as many pineapple cans as their father wished. 'He had a bench in the basement', Jack remembers. 'He had one of those multi-tools that could be a table saw, or you could turn it into a lathe. But mostly he used hand tools, draw blades and chisels. He was a true, mad inventor. I've seen him pick up a juice can, drive a nail through it and with a sparkle in his eye say, "I can use this!" Then he'd turn to my mother and demand, "I need a piece of string!" He was a Thomas Edison. He'd go round the house looking for things he could use, and whatever he found he'd make use of. I well remember him wrapping window screening and cellophane round those cans, and that was the start of the twin-coil dialyser.'

The disposable kidney stemmed from a visit by Kolff in 1955 to Philadelphia, where he'd seen a coil-type dialyser. It consisted of a coil of cellophane tubing wound together with the plastic mesh that is more commonly used as window screening to keep flies out of houses. When immersed in a bath of dialysing fluid, this simple device fulfilled all the requirements of an artificial kidney, provided the blood could flow through it and the dialysing fluid could be forced through the mesh screening so that it was in continuous moving contact with the cellophane – always a prime requirement of any artificial kidney.

What made this idea immediately attractive to Kolff was its obvious cheapness. He recognised that the used fruit juice can was all that was needed to provide a base on which the coil could be wound. 'I would have preferred a beer can, because there are more of them,' he says, 'but they're smaller than a juice can and so the resistance to the flow of blood would have been higher. If I used the next-sized can up, it would be a gallon can, which would have been too big because it would have needed too much blood to fill it. A fruit juice can was just right.' He added up the cost of items bought at a hardware store and reckoned his fruit juice can kidney cost a fraction over sixteen dollars. Now, he thought, with such a simple and cheap machine, dialysis would be available world-wide. Together, he and Watschinger published their ideas.

Pleased with their new artificial kidney, he took it to Abbott Laboratories, an emerging big player in the field of medical equipment. After six months he had heard nothing, so he wrote, 'If you don't give me a reply now, I'll take it somewhere else.' As a result Kolff was invited to give a presentation before the board of directors at which they applauded the machine and showed great enthusiasm. It was short-lived, though, for that night, word came through that they had decided against developing the idea. Eleven months later they were to change their minds and offered Kolff another invitation to talk. He didn't give them a second chance. 'I didn't see any point in that.'

Kolff had taken his invention elsewhere, to Baxter, another major player in the world of medical machinery. Here he found a warmer welcome, in particular from a Mr Graham who was intrigued by Kolff's idea. 'They immediately accepted,' Kolff remembers, 'but I was a little dismayed when they gave it to another engineer to develop. He was a nice man, but he made numerous variations on the theme of my juice can dialyser and we brought them all together to test them alongside each other, his against mine. We spent a whole day testing one after the other and he kept telling us how much better his was for the improvements he'd made. I thought the men from Baxter looked unconvinced, and my technician overheard the chief man from Baxter lean across to the engineer and say, "I think we'll do it Kolff's way."'

Within a year, Baxter's Travenol division had built 184 working artificial kidneys and thus started one of their great commercial successes. Over the years it must have contributed millions to their profits – and it still does to this day. Kolff, with no patent ever having been filed, has received not a penny.

In the time it took Baxter to bring the first commercially available kidneys into operation, Kolff had moved on and left them standing. He had invented yet another kidney, this time an even cheaper one which gave him even more satisfaction. Dr Holzenbein had discovered a new material which could be used to keep the cellophane coils apart; it was a kind of woven webbing, not unlike the material used to make potato sacks, and it could replace the window screening used in the twin-coil dialyser. Armed with the webbing and cellophane, Kolff reasoned, there was no reason why patients should not build their own dialysers at home, if they wanted. In fact, he went so far as to design a winding machine for them to use, and in doing so invented what might be called the world's first DIY dialyser. As with all such machines, the important principle is that the blood and the dialysing fluid should be in continuous moving contact, but how to achieve that on a domestic scale?

The answer lay in a common domestic appliance – a washing machine. Kolff saw that if the hand-wound twin-coil dialyser were placed in the washing machine, and it was filled with dialysing fluid instead of soapy water, the motion caused by the action of the washing machine would fulfil all the requirements of a dialysis machine. Tubes would carry the blood from the patient to the coil, which would be immersed in the washing machine containing the dialysing fluid. The whole apparatus could easily stand next to a bed. The action of the washing machine's paddle would ensure the necessary fluid contact between the solution and the membrane. He judged Maytag as being the best machine for the purpose, and proudly announced that for a cost of only $265 a month, which included the cellophane and all the dialysing salts, any patient could be taught to 'roll their own'.

There was one problem. Kolff remembers, 'One day, a lawyer from the Maytag company came into my office. I remember him because one leg was shorter than the other, and as soon as I saw him I knew there was trouble. He pointed out that if one of my patients died while connected to one of his washing machines, then the nuisance value of any lawsuit would be $22,000, a lot of money then. He warned me that Maytag were not in that kind of business, and dealers had been instructed not to supply me with them. So instead I bought them on the quiet, like dealing with the black market. What else could I do?'

Soon the Maytag problem was behind him when he discovered an even better – and cheaper – container for the dialysing fluids. He learnt that NASA had a considerable supply of surplus missile nose-cones. As a fierce opponent of nuclear proliferation, redirecting this surplus from the hands of weapon-makers into the more constructive realm of life-saving pleased him greatly. So the 'nose-cone dialyser' was his next invention. 'The nose-cones made wonderful tanks. I think I sent almost thirty patients home with nose-cones. The only problem with it was that it was *too* cheap. No company would produce these machines commercially because there would be so little profit for them. It was a very sad thing. The nose-cone dialyser became an orphan.'

Not all of Kolff's efforts at the Cleveland Clinic were directed towards the invention of artificial organs, and he took considerable steps into the world of more orthodox research, although typically he chose cutting-edge medicine and surgery. In the late 1950s, at a time when the Cleveland Clinic was opposed to the idea of the revolutionary new technique of kidney transplantation, Kolff seized upon it as a life-saver for those patients for whom dialysis was not a solution. The amount of time a patient could spend on dialysis was still limited by the number of occasions the tubes could be inserted into veins and arteries. With repeated dialysis it was easy for doctors to run out of access points. That problem was only solved in the early 1960s by Belding Scribner's invention of what became known as the Scribner shunt. This was a U-shaped tube, permanently installed between an artery and a vein, so that the kidney machine could be plugged into it and unplugged as required. It meant that repeated dialysis, for a lifetime if necessary, became a possibility.

This remained in the future, and Kolff believed transplantation was the only solution for patients who were suffering end-stage renal failure. Towards the end of 1954, at the Peter Bent Brigham Hospital in Boston, John Merrill performed the first successful human kidney transplantation by taking a kidney from one identical twin and giving it to his sick brother. This avoided any rejection problems, since the tissues of both donor and recipient were perfectly matched. Although this would be a highly unlikely occurrence in everyday practice, the success of the operation proved for the first time that transplantation was a real possibility.

A few years later, when Kolff decided that kidney transplantation was a technique the Cleveland Clinic should help perfect, he found himself yet again talking to a brick wall – otherwise well known to him as the Cleveland medical establishment. 'They were mortally opposed to transplantation. I had a young resident go round the hospital authorities to get their view, and they all said, "We can wait. Then, if it is later proven to work, we can get on the bandwagon."'

Kolff was no jumper on the backs of other people's bandwagons, much preferring to be the driver. Ignoring any opposition, he teamed up with a first-rate surgeon, Gene Poutos, and decided to employ the tactic which had worked so well for Bailey, the heart surgeon, when he wanted to prove that his technique involving the double-gloved hand with the concealed blade could be used to correct defects in mitral valves. Bailey had effectively run so fast that the hospital authorities had been unable to keep up with him to prevent him performing further operations: Kolff decided to do the same. 'We agreed we would do six kidney transplantations in rapid succession. We would do them so fast that they couldn't stop us.' But what Kolff also recognised about Bailey's approach was that it was only his *third* patient who survived. Had Bailey performed only one operation, it would have been judged a total failure, but when he had a surviving patient to prove it worked his technique was hailed as a breakthrough.

Kolff took six ill patients and removed both their kidneys (he believed at the time that the natural kidney might adversely affect the implanted organ). The donors were all living family members. Once the operations had been completed and the patients were well recovered, Kolff attended a staff meeting at which medical policy was discussed, and took the opportunity to parade all six thriving patients before the entire staff of the Cleveland Clinic. 'Those who had been against us had no other choice than to congratulate us. Of course, they tried to get back at us with a vengeance, but they couldn't stop us after that.'

Some six weeks later the first patient, a young lady, started to reject the implanted kidney. Kolff believes that if he and Poutos had been allowed to perform only one operation, which would have been on that young woman, they would have been stopped immediately, the girl's fate proving that transplantation did not work. But because the other five continued to thrive, Kolff and Poutos were praised for their skills.

Despite the pressures of hospital politics, nothing seemed to take the edge off Kolff's mind, for if he was not announcing yet another invention of his own, he was creating an atmosphere in which others could bend their minds to new techniques, to novel ways of replicating the functions of failing body organs. Kolff remembers coming into his laboratory one day to find Stephen Topaz and Spyros Moulopoulos playing with what appeared to be no more than a long, thin balloon connected to a pump which caused it to inflate and deflate roughly in the rhythm of a natural heartbeat. Even more curious was what happened when they inserted it into a working model of the human circulation, which Kolff used to test his ideas for artificial hearts and oxygenators. This unlikely device was to become the intra-aortic balloon pump, which is regularly used world-wide and in at least 100,000 patients annually in the USA. It consists of a balloon attached to the end of a catheter which is inserted into the femoral artery at the groin, from where it is threaded up the body and into the aorta, the largest artery in the body. Its method of operation is astonishingly simple. Between heartbeats, the long slender balloon is inflated. The effect of this is to act as an auxiliary pump and chase any blood which lies ahead of it out of the aorta. Before the heart makes its next contraction, the balloon collapses. When the heart then contracts, less effort is required because the aorta is empty and the ailing heart finds it has little work to do in filling it. Kolff is 'proud that I did not terminate this project which most department heads would have done at the time because it seemed such a crazy idea'.

Meanwhile, crazy ideas were becoming real ones. The *wearable* artificial kidney emerged from Kolff's laboratory, the work largely of Steve Jacobsen. To general astonishment kidney patients were able to take holidays by joining a 'Dialysis In Wonderland' programme run by a travel company; this gave them unprecedented freedom, to the extent that Kolff remembers a wearable dialyser functioning perfectly well while the patient was paddling a raft down the Colorado River.

Then in December 1957 Kolff, working with Tet Akutsu, kept a dog alive for ninety minutes with an artificial heart, its natural heart having been removed. So convinced did he become after this experiment that it would be possible to implant an artificial heart in people, that he published a booklet. He began his introduction thus: 'Perhaps the most dramatic of all research efforts is that which is now being directed towards the development of an artificial heart to replace a diseased heart. This challenge, which is as exciting as any throughout the entire range of science, is enormously complex, but the goal is feasible; the problems are not insuperable.'

However, he was also to note some time later: 'I have no doubt that someone else may be the first to implant an artificial heart or ventricle in a human being, but the first will not necessarily be the best, nor will it necessarily meet the minimum criteria that must be established for long-term artificial organs. We will implant a device only when we are satisfied that the patient can live a comfortable and reasonably normal life, unimpeded by the man-made heart in his chest.'

It reads like Kolff's declaration of war on the problems that were about to beset him.

11
REPLACING THE HEART AND SOUL

By the mid-1960s Kolff was becoming recognised world-wide and was dubbed 'the father of artificial organs'. His expertise in the field was unmatched, and his development of the artificial kidney was finally appreciated as the breakthrough Kolff always believed it would be. There was no longer any reason for him to confine himself to the Cleveland Clinic.

In a typically single-minded act he took a cut in salary to move to the University of Utah in 1967. Every penny it cost him was worth it, for at last he had found somewhere he was truly welcome and where his inventive intellect would be allowed to roam free, even though the university authorities warned him there was little cash to subsidise his inventions. He made enquiries, asking where the best regional medicine programme in the whole of the USA was to be found. There was no doubt, it was in Salt Lake City. A bioengineering programme had been established here in the late 1950s by the eminent Dr Homer Warner, a medical computing pioneer. As the university authorities predicted, the arrival of the 'father of artificial organs' as the new director of the department brought a flood of applications from researchers, students and engineers who wanted to work alongside Kolff.

'I remember going to the university in Salt Lake City,' he remembers, 'it was so restful. There was snow on the mountains and the sun shone on them. Fast-running rivers of clear water rushed down the main street.' He was clearly smitten with the place, and a few days after that first visit he went back to Salt Lake, this time with Janke, who had found a house overlooking a mountain valley – they bought it even before Kolff had signed a contract with the university. 'From the very beginning I knew I was going to be happy there. Utah State Governor Rampton even shook my hand in welcome!'

Even so, Kolff was again obliged to work in conditions he describes as 'eccentric', in wooden buildings – former Second World War barracks – at the back of the university. But the job came with a warning: 'They told me they had no objections to accepting government money, unlike Cleveland, but that any money I needed for research I would have to raise myself. I didn't mind this. They said they would help me if I wished to start a company, which I did, and all my co-workers got shares at a penny each, and six months later those shares were worth a dollar.'

The barracks became his laboratory, and although it was not equipped or suitable for the treatment of human patients, it was more than adequate for Kolff's development work, which involved as much engineering as medicine and surgery. Indeed, Kolff was to engineer for himself a unique position in Salt Lake City, for not only was he a member of the department of surgery, but also of the departments of internal medicine, engineering and research. As a colleague remarked, 'In that position, no one could stop him.' He was now fifty-six years old, which some might consider to be a little late in life to be opening a new chapter – that is, if they didn't know Kolff.

For his assistants and fellow researchers he was forced to look outside the American medical community, remarking that, 'The majority of people who finish medical school have a $60,000 dollar debt, and residents are paid very little. Most of them simply couldn't afford to work for me unless they had other appointments. So the majority of my co-workers came from the Far East.' But some came from Europe, in particular Horst Klinkmann, who has the distinction of being the only surviving pupil of two kidney inventors, Kolff and the Swede, Alwall. Klinkmann had gained his medical qualifications at the University of Rostock, then part of Communist-controlled East Germany, and had taken with him a replica of Alwall's artificial kidney, making Rostock the only place in either East or West Germany where dialysis could be performed. Like all pioneers of kidney dialysis, Klinkmann was apparently the object of deep suspicion. 'I remember a very severe German professor to whom I was trying to explain dialysis and the benefits of it. He turned to me and said, "Young man, stop talking about *killing* our patients." Those doctors who went along with dialysis did so because they believed the great advantage of it was that it would put people out of their misery with great speed.'

Klinkmann had come to Kolff's attention because of his pioneering work in the dialysis of young children, and the first invitation to work alongside Kolff came in 1962 while he was still in Cleveland. Klinkmann remembers, 'I was asked to go to the farm and was very disappointed by the visit. All I was asked to do was drive the tractor but I wanted to talk about science, but I don't think we spoke a word on the subject all weekend.'

It was some years later that Klinkmann eventually joined Kolff in Salt Lake City after an urgent phone call which began, 'Can you come in three months?' For a doctor to travel from a Communist country to work in America was unusual, and Kolff was instrumental in fixing visas and writing references – to the extent that when Klinkmann arrived at US immigration to have his papers examined, the officer remarked, 'You're the first highly desirable

Communist we've had through here.' His visa was duly stamped, and he was through.

Klinkmann agrees that 'Kolff was much happier in Salt Lake City. In Cleveland he was seen as exotic and demanding, an immigrant with ideas, and a poor diplomat too. They were happy to take all the glory that came from his work, but all the time they were looking down on him. His great talent? That was to bring together all the disciplines of medicine and engineering. He was the first to do that.'

Kolff found himself the director of a department which had become largely defunct, with no funding other than that which he could raise by his own efforts, and with a formidable agenda which included further improvements to the artificial kidney and the heart/lung machine, the perfection of the artificial heart and development of the artificial eye, ear and arm. At the end of this list Kolff added an enigmatic and optimistic 'etc.'

Like many scientists before him, Kolff came face to face with the daunting prospect of raising money to fund his research. He remembers, 'I went to the Mount Sinai Hospital in Cleveland to learn the new cost analysis programme that estimated every sponge, every needle and every bottle of saline. It was horrible. But I did my best and wrote a proposal to the Public Health Service for a wind-it-yourself artificial kidney, and we got the contract which established the dialysis centre in Utah.'

By 1973 Kolff had created a small kingdom in Utah, bringing together technicians, engineers, designers and surgeons, and in that year he published a prospectus for the Division of Artificial Organs. At first glance it reads not unlike a work of science fiction, for here appears to be the blueprint for the bionic man; a creature created in the laboratory whose organs are not fashioned out of human tissues, but made of plastics and metal. It is not driven by impulses through nerve fibres but by electric currents sent through copper wires. In this ambitious, if not fanciful, manifesto, we read of his plans for cardiac assist devices and total heart replacement: 'In coming years we will perfect artificial hearts with power sources outside the body to the point where they will become clinically applicable.' A page further on, we read of the 'atomically powered heart driven by a plutonium-based radioactive source'. Already they are using computer graphics to measure blood flows and predict likely turbulence in artificial hearts, and we are told that the microcircuit laboratory is the 'most strongly staffed in the United States' and declares 'we can send signals into the brain such as will be used for the artificial eye and the artificial ear, or derive signals from the brain, such as from the motor cortex to enervate a paralysed limb'. It was such an imaginative and bold agenda that even a fire in 1973 failed to halt Kolff and his team. He wrote, 'On May the 5th, our main building was burned out. It contained our operating rooms, heart testing rooms, mould rooms and some of our most expensive equipment. Our collection of artificial hearts since 1957 was lost. However, our newest and most promising heart was salvaged.' The heart that survived the fire was to make headlines like no artificial organ had done before or since. It was the Jarvik heart.

A point of clarification is needed here. Although the heart is known and identified with its co-designer Robert Jarvik, it might equally accurately be described as Kolff's. It was Kolff's practice to christen devices after the researcher conducting the development work at the time. Kolff wrote: 'When somebody in our Division of Artificial Organs works on an artificial heart, it carries his name for easy identification. Thus, we have had Akutsu hearts, Norton hearts, Nose's giant atria, Lyman hearts, Donovan hearts,

Kwan Gett hearts, Unger hearts, and Jarvik hearts. The man who worked on the heart published it under his name as first author. The only thing we have not had is a Kolff heart.' He did not worry about the name: it was the device that mattered to him. In fact, after the successful implantation of the world's first artificial heart Kolff publicly thanked 247 co-workers – of which Jarvik was but one.

Kolff and Jarvik understood each other well technically. A former medical student in Bologna, Jarvik came to Kolff's laboratory looking for work. Kolff remembers him as a good inventor, best at taking ideas forward, happier at developmental rather than conceptual work, and 'good to work with'. Jarvik had many of the talents needed of a medical inventor, for apart from an enthusiasm for medicine, he had studied architecture, which led to an interest in three-dimensional art, and he had already invented a surgical stapling machine by the time he was discovered by Kolff. Kolff enjoyed the young man's company, and 'treated him like a son', as one associate described the relationship. But it was to develop into a working relationship which some considered too close. 'Yes, we had a father/son relationship,' Kolff admits, 'and I was warned about that by some colleagues. In the end, they were right.'

If Kolff's attempt to replicate the function of the kidney was audacious, then the idea of building an artificial heart which could be permanently implanted and would sustain life was on the verge of playing God. Kolff knew this. Indeed, it had been suggested to him that this was one step too far, and that the heart was the symbol of love, the repose of the soul, the source of affection and understanding – and to remove it and replace it with a crude mechanical device was verging on the unacceptable.

Philosophical arguments apart, the sheer mechanics of it were awesome. The facts are these: the heart beats 100,000 times a day, making for 35 million beats a year which, added up over an average lifetime, makes 2.5 billion muscular contractions. The purpose of these is to move the 5.6 litres of blood that your body contains through your entire circulation system three times every minute. In one day your blood will have travelled 12,000 miles – or four times across the width of the United States. If you want a more potent image, then the amount of blood pumped by the heart in a lifetime will fill three supertankers. All this from an organ the size of two of your fists. If you want to feel the force with which it works, then you should take hold of a tennis ball and squeeze it hard until it gives: that is the amount of energy required for each contraction of the heart. And Kolff thought he could devise a machine which would do that, and keep on doing it, never missing a beat.

There had been work on the artificial heart before Kolff's. Dr Paul Winchell had patented a design back in the 1950s and was persuaded to donate the patent to the University of Utah for further research. Kolff meanwhile had continued with experimental implantations of artificial hearts into calves, and had achieved survival rates of up to forty-eight hours, during which time the animals were 'awake and alert'. However, the major problem – the tendency of the blood to form destructive clots – was not solved until the discovery that forms of polyurethane plastics not only were able to sustain the repeated mechanical demands of an artificial heart, but also showed themselves not to cause the formation of clots. Another benefit was that this material could be moulded into a seamless sac. As a result, survival rates dramatically increased to over a hundred days. This revealed other problems, in particular the tendency for tissue to grow across the joint between the arteries and the artificial heart, leading to loss of efficiency as the inlets and outlets narrowed. This called for a rethink of the attachment technique.

The drive unit which delivered power to the artificial heart was no simple matter either. As the journal of the American Society of Artificial Internal Organs recorded in 1959: 'The pumping action of the mammalian heart would seem at first to be one of the simplest functions of an internal organ to imitate with a man-made device.' But the more research was invested in the development of the artificial heart, the more that view was to be proved wrong. Should the heart be powered by solenoids, or small electric motors? Could they be made small enough to implant, and if so precisely where would they fit? Could the power supply ever be made small enough, and, most importantly, could one ever be devised which could respond to the body's ever-changing demands for blood, as in exercise or mere movement? One fundamental point, which Kolff realised early on, was that any artificial heart, like a human heart, must obey Starling's Law, the work of a British physiologist working at the end of the nineteenth century. Put very simply, the input pressure of the blood determines the output of the heart. A successful artificial heart would have to obey that law. It was far from being a simple pump.

The Kolff heart was not the first to be tested on a human being. That distinction goes to the Liotta heart, implanted by Denton Cooley on 4 April 1969. Cooley was among the first surgeons in the USA to perform a successful heart transplant. At the time he was working in the surgery department of Baylor University, of which Michael DeBakey was head. DeBakey, a personal adviser to almost every American president of the last fifty years, is a surgeon of almost mythical status. According to his biography he has operated on 'heads of state, princes and celebrities, as well as paupers', although he was absent when Cooley performed the artificial implant.

The patient was a 47-year-old man, Haskell Karp, who had been operated on to repair a left ventricular aneurysm, but could not be weaned off cardiopulmonary bypass. The artificial heart that Cooley implanted was the invention of Domingo Liotta, who had worked with both Cooley and DeBakey and, briefly, Kolff, but its career was a brief if famous one. The heart supported Karp for only sixty-four hours, but during that time renal failure developed. When a heart became available for transplant the patient was already in a poor condition, and after transplant survived only a further thirty-two hours. The Liotta heart was never used again.

Meanwhile Kolff's team of 'heart boys', as he called his gang of designers, edged closer to the day when they would be able to test a heart of their invention on a human patient. Kolff's first task was to find a surgeon willing to risk his reputation on the implantation of such a highly experimental device. Few were forthcoming, sensing the small possibility of glory but the much greater potential for widespread condemnation. William DeVries had been a student in Kolff's department from the start, and was the only surgeon Kolff could entice to perform the operation. Merely gaining permission to do so took twenty-two months of negotiation – which came to an abrupt halt when, to Kolff's horror, the question was asked, 'What if a suitable patient comes forward who can't afford to pay for the procedure?' The question of the patient being able to pay the bill at the end of an historic artificial heart implantation was never high on Kolff's agenda, so he spent his valuable time persuading a charitable foundation in New York to underwrite the cost of the operation to the tune of $50,000 if the patient did not have the means.

Meanwhile Kolff's son Jack, now a heart surgeon, had been performing implantations on brain-dead cadavers, with family permission, in order to arrive at some conclusion as to how the artificial heart could best be placed. At first glance it might seem obvious that the human heart would simply be removed and the device dropped into the cavity. It proved far less simple than that, for the human heart is placed neatly between the spine and the breastbone for maximum protection. But for a larger, artificial heart, there often wasn't the room. As Jack remarked, 'You've got to squeeze 'em in, you know. It's not always easy, quite a challenge. I didn't always get the bodies I wanted. They came in all shapes and sizes.' Not only was the device larger, it was also less pliable than the heart it was replacing. Yet after five operations, Jack knew precisely where it should be placed. This was, of course, vital knowledge for the surgeon who was to perform the first implant in a patient, but to Kolff's regret Jack's valuable experience was never put to good use.

DeVries knew a cardiologist who, by chance, mentioned that a patient of his might be suitable for the implantation of an artificial heart. He was Barney Clark, a 61-year-old dentist from Seattle, for whom a human transplant was not an option because of his age. 'He was an intelligent man,' says Kolff, 'who knew he was going to die. In fact, it was almost certain that he would die the night I met him.' The question of the artificial heart had already been raised, and they discussed whether he might consent to the procedure. It was explained to him that it called for considerable courage, and that the outcome was far from certain. Now he had to decide. The only guarantee was that by the morning he would be dead if no action was taken. As DeVries put it to Clark, 'We don't gain much by waiting.'

A few evenings before, Barney Clark had been taken down to the barn at the back of the hospital where the calves lived. Some of them were being kept alive by artificial hearts, and they were not just alive but fit and well too. Clark looked at them and said, 'They can't speak, but they sure look better than I feel.' The consent form enabling the groundbreaking operation to proceed ran to fourteen pages. Barney Clark signed it.

He was made ready for the operation, and the artificial heart, supplied by Kolff's company, Kolff Associates, was prepared.

The operation took place on 2 December 1982 at the University Hospital in Salt Lake City. It was a huge media event. Crowds of reporters and observers descended on the hospital; helicopters hovered over the hospital grabbing television pictures. It was top news on television stations around the world, for the journalists were quick to recognise that this was totally unlike Cooley's implantation: this time it was not an operation to act as a life-saving bridge until a donor heart could be found. This was to be Barney Clark's heart for as long as he lived.

While the operation took place, Kolff waited at home, containing his natural inclination to be in the operating room. 'I just sat at home. There was nothing I could do. If I wanted to know how he was getting on, I used to ring a reporter.' The day after the operation, Kolff went to see Barney Clark. 'He looked good, really good. And did for several days after that. I made several recommendations about his treatment, but they weren't taken up. Of course, he wasn't my patient.'

Soon, the press were clamouring to meet the inventor of this miraculous new device that was keeping Barney Clark alive. A press conference was convened in the hospital cafeteria. Kolff remembers, 'Jarvik always seemed to be on the front row. I didn't care if he got the credit. I'd talked to my team about what might happen, and I'd warned them that when the heart is implanted all the fame will go to the surgeon who puts it in. You don't know if your name will be mentioned, I told them. If you can't take that then you should look for another position. The consolation is that if the patient dies, then it's the surgeon who goes to prison. However, William DeVries, the surgeon, was always loyal, and if there was a group picture he ensured I was in it, and my staff too.' But it was Jarvik who became the hero of the day. The press reasoned that because the heart was called the Jarvik heart, the credit should go to him. They needed a single hero, not a whole team of technicians, and the presentable young Jarvik fitted the bill nicely.

The media remained totally unaware of what precisely had taken place in the operating room, and had they known they might have been less enthusiastic in reporting the procedure. In Kolff's view, there were a number of problems. First, a vital piece of equipment was missing – there was no membrane oxygenator. If anyone knew about the kind of heart/lung machine needed to keep Clark alive while the operation proceeded, then it was Kolff, for he had been partially instrumental in inventing it. Kolff, however, knew that a bubble oxygenator had been used instead. This would have been satisfactory in an operation of short duration, but in one which took seven-and-a-half hours the action of oxygen bubbling through the blood would do severe physical damage to the red cells, leading to possible renal failure. A membrane oxygenator was what was needed. Secondly, when the implantation was complete, a major problem presented itself. 'They couldn't close the chest', says Kolff. 'They'd put the heart in the wrong place and it was impossible to close the chest over it, so it had to be removed and put back in again.' Of course, Jack Kolff could have told them the correct positioning for he had done the experiments.

Nevertheless, Clark was alive after the lengthy operation and, as Kolff recorded, 'We learned that the artificial heart inside the chest did not hurt, that the noise from the drive system did not bother him, that he had not lost his considerable sense of humour, and that after the removal of his natural heart he still loved his family and wanted to serve his fellow humans. All the properties of the human mind that are really important are preserved.'

A few days later, however, it was a different story. Clark went into series of severe convulsions. To add to the complications, a mechanical valve failed and had to be replaced in a further operation. 'He shook like I've never seen a person shake before', Kolff remembers. 'So they gave him drugs, huge doses, to try to stop it until he was nearly comatose, but his arm still shook. At the time, they had no idea why.' Kolff has his own theory, but points out that Clark was not his patient and any advice he offered was usually ignored, especially his suggestion that Clark was being over-hydrated. 'I think they gave him a deadly overdose of theophylline, a muscle relaxant. Why the laboratory never detected it in the blood tests I shall never know. Possibly it was reported by its chemical name and not its commercial name, and wasn't spotted. A nephrologist recognised it later when someone went through the charts with a fine tooth comb. Because of the damage done by the bubble oxygenator, the kidneys had been severely weakened and they'd been unable to expel the overdose.'

Barney Clark lived for 112 days, and his death was recorded as being due to fulminating colitis. Despite reports that he suffered repeated strokes, Kolff and other sources insist no stroke took place, thus proving the heart did not manufacture blood clots. That alone was a significant advance.

Hindsight has been less than kind about the pioneering procedure carried out on Barney Clark. In the context of more recent work, it was reported that the problems of the

Jarvik 7 were that 'it ran on pulses of air that jolted Clark with every beat. The patient had to be tied to an external wind machine and have large hoses piercing his chest.' They added, 'It took Barney Clark 112 miserable days to die after being fitted with the Jarvik 7. Four months of suffering that included convulsions, kidney failure, respiratory problems, a wandering mind and, finally, multi-organ system failure.' In the aftermath of that débâcle, the *New York Times* nicknamed artificial heart research the 'Dracula of Modern Technology'. Kolff has a different memory. 'He had many problems, most of them nothing to do with the artificial heart, and for times he was very well. He told me his heart didn't bother him, and he expressly wished it not to be shut off.'

Perhaps it should be judged as less of a breakthrough and more of a significant experiment. It was indeed a long and slow death for Barney Clark, but there is no doubt that it was pivotal to the development of heart surgery.

Kolff's subsequent career changed too, and the course of it was dictated not by any weakening in his inventive skills, but, as Horst Klinkmann says, 'he was the greatest of inventors and the worst of businessmen'. His abiding belief throughout his entire career had been that none of his inventions should be beyond anyone's pocket. He'd taken his kidney machine and refined it until it could be constructed by the patients themselves using a juice can and window screening. Now he wanted artificial hearts to be cheap too, and easily built in hours rather than days.

Kolff had embraced the new technology of vacuum forming not only for its inherent cheapness but also for the reliability with which thin membranes could be made to close tolerances, without any danger of the pinholes created by conventional mould-forming methods. Kolff spent a year in Germany studying what he believed to be the ideal way to handle plastic in the production of artificial hearts. But Jarvik, now a key player in Kolff's company, was not convinced, even though it reduced the building time from eighteen days to just two, with a consequent massive reduction in cost. As a result Kolff resigned as chairman of Kolff Associates. It was an acrimonious end to Kolff's working relationship with Jarvik, about which he remains bitter.

Jack Kolff, however, was still keen on the development work, and applied to the all-powerful Food and Drugs Administration (FDA), to be allowed to undertake further implantations. Approval was not forthcoming. The price of the hearts, which they were now forced to buy from Jarvik, escalated in price. 'I tried to reason with Jarvik. I told him that we'd helped him, why didn't he help us? But he didn't.' Jack Kolff was unable to raise the $200,000 dollars needed to purchase the Jarvik hearts for live clinical trials, and instead turned to vacuum-formed artificial hearts – a technique developed and refined by his father. The vacuum-formed heart, though, was also in some difficulty. Without some experimental data on which to base a judgement, the FDA could not even consider giving approval for an implantation, so experiments on calves were carried out to prove that the heart could sustain the circulation for thirty days, which was the FDA's requirement. Jack Kolff explains: 'Having shown that the heart *did* work for thirty days, we terminated the experiment, thinking we had the data we needed. Then the FDA came back to us and said that the waiting time for transplants had increased and so they needed to see data beyond thirty days. We couldn't afford to start over again.' At the same time Jack Kolff was advised by his university that too much money had already been spent, and that he had three months to finish his research. Shortly afterwards, he took up private practice in Johnstown, Pennsylvania.

Kolff remembers, 'I retained a small laboratory in Salt Lake City with Steve Topaz and David Jones. There was no place for Jarvik. William DeVries went to Louisville. That was that.'

Forty years after Kolff had first connected his patients to his early kidney machines, nearly half a century after he had first observed the oxygenation of the blood as it flowed through his crude sausage skin dialyser, and realised that the same arterial connection that linked patient and kidney machine might provide an opportunity to attach an oxygenator, the artificial heart of which he had dreamed was effectively out of his hands, if not out of his thoughts.

12
'MY COLLABORATORS'

One morning, nearly sixty years after Kolff had pioneered the use of his artificial kidney and proved its value by indisputably saving a life, I stood with him in the entrance to the old Kampen Hospital. It is no longer an inspiring place. The windows are mostly boarded up, and those few that still show some glass have been either broken or left unwashed. The hospital where radical life-saving techniques were first developed is itself in its death throes.

The caretaker let us in through a padlocked side door, the main entrance being boarded up, and we wandered along the corridors, Kolff leading the way. The mosaic on the floor of the imposing entrance, complete with sweeping staircase, boasted that the hospital had been built in 1913. Kolff looked around, as at home in this setting as if it had been only a few short months since he last strode the corridors, his heels clicking across the marble floors warning nurses and patients that he was on his way. He flung his arms wide to embrace the lobby: '*Here* they all danced on my birthday. It was a very friendly atmosphere in this little hospital. I taught the nurses anatomy, which was good,' he chuckled, 'because it meant I had to relearn it!' An old photograph of the nursing staff showed what a proud and tidy bunch they were, dressed in blue uniforms with white aprons held up by crossed braces. 'One nurse', Kolff remembered, 'was a National Socialist [a Nazi supporter] but she never betrayed us. It was that sort of place.'

We came to Room 12a, the 'kidney room' in which the

later patients were dialysed. It was, in fact, Room 13, but Kolff thought this might make superstitious patients uneasy. He strolled in as if he were still a young doctor attending a patient, his face wearing a smile of recognition, of feeling at home. 'My machine was over there,' he pointed, then glanced at the floor, 'and sometimes the room was awash with blood and dialysing fluid and we put down bricks to use as stepping stones.' It was an unremarkable room for so much history.

We visited the old X-ray room, his office and the hospital wards, and then he said farewell to the place and closed the door behind him. Together we crossed a paved square to a statue that had been erected in his honour. The inscription simply read 'Fighter for Public Health'. Made of bronze, it is a bust from which his piercing eye stares across towards the very room where his invention took shape. The breast is modelled in the shape of a kidney: 'They made it look like a suit of armour,' said Kolff, 'to show that it was a fight. And they sculpted it so that it looked as though I had one hand tied behind my back, because of the war.'

For a man whose inventive mind has not been in the slightest blunted by the passing years, there was always going to be a question over his retirement. The notion that there might be a period of his life which was not consumed entirely with his lifetime's work has never entered his head. To switch off remains unimaginable to him. There cannot have been a morning of his adult life when he hasn't woken with a medical problem on his mind and reached for a solution. He was born with a brain that never wants to rest.

Later that day he attended the annual meeting of the Prof. W. Kolff Institute, conceived as a forum for a discussion of medical matters and their social implications. They had dedicated that year's meeting to a celebration of his ninetieth birthday. It was held in the city's theatre, and his old associates were there to honour him, and to shake his hand again. Bob van Noordwijk, once Kolff's young, studious and enthusiastic assistant, who became professor of pharmacology at the University of Utrecht, gave his reminiscences of the early experiments. Remembering Kolff, and the roller-coaster ride of hope and disappointment that accompanied the early attempts at dialysis, he remarked, 'If the kidney machine had been invented anywhere else but in Kampen, I think it would have got a lot more world-wide attention. Look at how Christiaan Barnard was celebrated for the first heart transplant. Kolff got none of that celebrity.' In Kampen, however, he remains a true hero. Alongside Bob and his surviving laboratory technicians, the new generation of doctors and surgeons stood to pay tribute to him.

As the conference commenced, Kolff, hard of hearing, frail of limb, but amazingly bright of eye and mind, took his place on the front row. He knew full well he was there to be celebrated, and those who know him well say that the sound of applause falls comfortably on his ears. He enjoys his star status, and of all his decorations there is one honour he always mentions first: 'In 1990 I was named by *Life* magazine as one of the hundred most important Americans of the twentieth century', but he quickly adds, 'Al Capone was on the list too, so we weren't all good guys.'

Dr John Jacobze, chairman of the Kolff Institute, a Kampen doctor and medical administrator whose father had given Kolff his first job in Kampen, reminded the conference that 'Kolff's accomplishments remain unparalleled and he truly began a new era of life-saving. He opened the bionic age. He is one of the living legends of medicine.'

Willem Kolff doesn't like death if it can be avoided, even of a hospital building, and on the morning we met he was fresh from addressing the Kampen City Council in an attempt to inspire them to preserve the old hospital as a museum to acknowledge its place in medical history. The hospital is now closed, and its proposed new use as a nursing home would involve the destruction of Room 12a, Kolff's famous kidney room. Behind the scenes he is lobbying local and national governments, and giving interviews to Dutch newspapers, 'to save the old hospital'. With hardly any less energy than he applied to the seemingly intractable problems of bringing together sausage skins and Ford water pump couplings, he is now fighting to save the battlefield on which he won his most famous victory.

His old colleague of forty-one years, Horst Klinkmann, took to the stage at the conference and reminded us of Kolff's simple declaration made over fifty years ago that, 'If a man knows the structure and function of one of the parts of his body, he should be able to build it. No hurdle was too high for Kolff. But alas, he's made other companies very rich. That's the fate of the pioneer. However, he is truly the father of artificial organs, of that there is no doubt.' Afterwards, Klinkmann said to me, privately, that he thought Kolff had always been misjudged. 'His opposition to the Vietnam War, and his membership of Physicians Against Nuclear War cost him the Nobel Prize, I am sure of that. Whenever he gave a public lecture, or a speech, he always added political comments at the end, and that didn't go down well.'

Although Kolff retired, formally, as the director of the department of biomedical engineering in Salt Lake City in 1986, life has hardly been quiet since. Until 1997, by which time he was eighty-six years old, he held the post of research professor and director of the laboratory that bears his name at the University of Utah. Occasionally a medical breakthrough born out of Kolff's early work still occurs and makes headline news across the world. During the writing of this book, it was reported that scientists had successfully constructed an artificial eye which would give sight to the totally blind. A couple of weeks after the news appeared, a note from Kolff arrived in the post reminding me that the early work on this was done by him and William Dobelle back in the late 1960s. Kolff says, 'I remember Dobelle stepping into my office and saying he wanted to work on the artificial eye. We did some research on what blind people wanted, but surprisingly reading wasn't high on the list, except for the sign that says "Men" or "Women". But they wanted to be able to walk around without bumping into things or other people.'

In 1968 research had shown that electrical stimulation of parts of the brain could produce the sensation of seeing a point of light. Other researchers had shown that similar stimulation of the acoustic nerve in the cochlea of the ear could give rise to a hearing sensation in totally deaf people. On that scientific basis, Dobelle and Kolff pressed ahead, convinced that the artificial eye and ear were a real possibility. The legacy of their early enthusiasm bore fruit when, in 1999, Dobelle finally demonstrated the application of the artificial eye in a totally blind man from Brooklyn. To prove the efficiency of the device – which, to put it at its simplest, uses microcircuitry (developed in Kolff's laboratory) to send impulses down wires patched to the brain – the blind man was able to navigate his way around tables and chairs deliberately placed to trip him up. Kolff remembers of the early experiments, 'When the first blind man reported that he could indeed see light, it was a profound emotional experience for all of us. Some, including myself, cried.' Similarly, as a result of work to produce an artificial ear, he remembers 'A Baptist minister who had been deaf flushed the toilet ten times in quick succession because he so loved the sound of rushing water.'

These are brief glimpses of Kolff's legacy, achieved not only by his own hands and in his own head, but also through the inspiration and encouragement he gave to others who came to work alongside him. In describing Kolff's contribution to the artificial eye programme, Dobelle wrote, 'To the best of my memory, Kolff never admonished people for "thinking the unorthodox thoughts". It was, he says, "the unwritten law of his laboratory".'

He also gives an insight into the way Kolff formed his team, for Dobelle was only twenty-six years old, did not have a doctoral degree, and was working at the time as the director of the Maryland Republican Party, although for seven years he had studied the physiology of vision at Johns Hopkins University, Baltimore. Dobelle writes, 'Kolff rarely hired people with conventional credentials, and he recently reiterated to me that "the fact is people with conventional credentials never wanted to work with me anyway".'

'There are many aspects of artificial vision which cannot be explained on the basis of cellular neurophysiology', Dobelle continues. 'When questioned about similar mysteries related to the artificial kidney, Kolff once stated with some heat that, "If I worried about such things, I would still be studying ion transport in cellophane membranes, and I would never have built the artificial kidney."'

Kolff was never happier than when fabricating devices with his own hands, although the word 'device' is anathema to him, for he learnt early in his career that as soon as an idea is described as a 'device' then it is regarded as a worthless gadget, and never taken seriously after that.

To prove the point that he has not lost one ounce of his love for invention, Kolff took to the stage of Kampen Theatre. First, he thanked all of his co-workers throughout his entire career, especially applauding the lifelong support of his first assistant, Bob van Noordwijk, and his son Jack, also a speaker on that morning. Then, with the panache of a true showman, he asked the audience if they wanted him to show them how to make an artificial heart out of an apple. They roared that they did. He picked up an apple from the table and sliced it in half with a penknife that he pulled from his pocket. He placed the apple, cut side down on the table, and placed two metal bottle tops on it, a large one for the inflow and a smaller one for what he described as the outflow. Over the top of the apple, complete with its bottle tops, he placed a plastic film, like a slice of ready cut cheese. 'This is all you need', he declared, as the audience followed every move like children at a party mesmerised by a magician. Over the apple he placed a heat lamp; beneath the apple was a grid below which was placed a small domestic vacuum cleaner. Slowly the plastic (which he explained was a kind of polythene called pellethane) softened and drooped around the apple to enclose it completely. By now the audience was enthralled. Kolff explained that a draught of cool air sets the plastic and then it can be peeled away. You have half a heart.

And so it goes on. A second sheet of plastic is vacuum-formed around the other half of the apple. A diaphragm is moulded to fit between the two halves, and flap valves are provided at the inlets and outlets. Finally space is provided for a motor that can pump 7 litres of blood a minute – and suddenly, out of an apple and a couple of sheets of plastic, you have an artificial heart.

Kolff did not demonstrate this entirely for his or his audience's amusement. It was to prove that artificial organ production can be cheap and simple, and that there is fun in invention. 'I remember students coming to my laboratory, and they all wanted to study blood flow, or something academic like that. But I insisted that everyone had to have a project, and make something with their own hands. That is what it's all about.'

His evangelism is undimmed. From his case he pulled out yet another artificial heart, its ventricles held together with Velcro. He ripped them apart, held them in the air and declared, 'People only a day from certain death have been implanted with these and within a couple of days are walking round asking for breakfast.'

He took one question from the audience: are you a stubborn man? 'No,' he replied, 'but I'm determined. I'm not very intelligent, but I do not accept that something can't be done!' To thunderous applause he left the stage.

He no longer lives with his wife Janke. You might think that a marriage which had lasted sixty years would endure a few more, but Kolff admits that his inability to give up his work completely may have been difficult for her to tolerate. She agrees. I asked his neighbour, Diana Carroll, if at home he showed any signs of declaring himself retired. She shook her head. 'He goes over to the local hardware store, and they all help him and they're very fond of him. He comes back with plastic pipes. In the sheltered housing where we both live there's an arts and crafts room and he took over one of the tables. Then another became available, and he took over that. I've seen him go shopping for kettles. He says he's working on a new method of dialysis.'

I challenged Kolff with this and instantly his eyes sparkled. 'The pipes are for something I dreamt up one night. After all these years I still wake up with new ideas.' He opens his briefcase and produces a prototype for a device to assist the left ventricle of a failing heart. His model is made from transparent polythene hose-pipe, glued together with whatever the craft room could provide. 'I first thought of this in 1973,' he declares, 'but nobody followed it up. There are 200,000 people in the USA alone who are living an unsatisfactory life. This could solve their problem.'

And now his ideas have taken him one step further, and

he feels the wearable artificial lung is now a real possibility. In another of his dawn wakings, a memory returned of an experiment conducted first in 1973 and again in 1983. The details do not matter here, but that he can still take an idea of twenty years ago and fashion from it something as unlikely as an artificial lung, which the wearer will put on like a waistcoat, proves that this is no ordinary mind at work. A million and a half patients are dialysed every year. Doubtless each one of those would testify to the worth of Kolff's ceaseless mind.

After the conference the old team from Kampen Hospital gathered in a restaurant. Bob van Noordwijk was there, so too Willy Eskes and Mieneke van der Leij. And when the dinner was over they helped Kolff to his feet and together they took a stroll down the main street of Kampen. Kolff spied an ice-cream shop, and soon a queue was forming with him at the head of it. With ice-creams in their fists, this band of elderly pioneers made their way through the town, laughing, joking, remembering. And in a gesture of deep and genuine affection for them all, Kolff flung his arms wide to embrace them and declared, 'These were my *true* collaborators!'

APPENDIX

CURRICULUM VITAE

Willem Johann Kolff

Born	14 February 1911 in the Netherlands
Citizenship	United States (1956); moved to the United States in 1950
Education	*1938* University of Leiden medical school, Holland, MD
	1946 University of Groningen (Summa cum Laude) PhD
Positions	*1940–50* internal medicine, Kampen, the Netherlands
	1950 Cleveland Clinic
	1967–86 Director of the Institute for Biomedical Engineering
	1967–86 Director of the Division of Artificial Organs, University of Utah, Salt Lake City
	1982–97 Distinguished Professor of Medicine and Surgery, Research Professor of Engineering and Director of W.J. Kolff's Laboratory, department of surgery, University of Utah, Salt Lake City
Awards	Total: 101 National and International Awards
	Commandeur in the Order of Oranje-Nassau
	12 honorary doctorates
	1964 Cameron Prize of the University of Edinburgh, Scotland

1972 The Harvey Prize from Technion
1974 Orden de mayo al Meriton en el Grado de Gran Official, the highest civilian award from the Argentine government
1986 The Japan Prize
1990 Counted as one of the 'hundred most important Americans of the Century' in the special autumn issue of *Life* magazine

Publications More than 600

Notes on Sources

Much of the content of this book was derived from transcripts of tapes made by Professor Kolff and relies largely on his memory of events supported by interviews with those who worked with him. A detailed account of the development of Kolff's artificial kidney has been written by his close associate, Professor Jacob (Bob) van Noordwijk *Dialysing for Life*, published by Kluwer Academic Publisher, in both Dutch and English. Students of the history of dialysis will do no better than the recent *The history of the treatment of renal failure by dialysis* by Professor J. Stewart Cameron, published by Oxford University Press (ISBN 0-19-851547-2).

A catalogued collection of Kolff's published papers and some personal material is held by the manuscripts division of the University of Utah, Marriott Library, Salt Lake City, Utah.

Kolff published three important papers relating to the development of the artificial kidney:

1: 'The artificial kidney: a dialyser with a great area', written by W.J. Kolff with the co-operation of Sister M. ter Welle, Miss A.J.W. van der Leij, E.C. van Dijk and J. van Noordwijk. This was published in a shortened form in English and French.
2: 'De kunstmatige nier [The artificial kidney]' – his thesis with which he obtained his doctorate in medicine at the University of Groningen on 16 January 1946.
3: 'New ways of treating uraemia' by W.J. Kolff with the assistance of J. van Noordwijk, P.S.M. Kop, N.K.M. van de Leeuw and A.M. Joekes.

Medical researchers will find a wealth of material relating to the development of artificial organs through established medical libraries, in particular the journals published by the ASAIO, the American Society for Artificial Internal Organs.

The Barney B. Clark Collection (1910–84) provides information on the development of the Jarvik 7 artificial heart, and the implantation of this heart into Dr Barney Bailey Clark, the first authorised recipient. This collection is held by the Marriott Library at the University of Utah.

The careers of distinguished heart surgeons Denton A. Cooley and Michael E. DeBakey are described by the Texas Heart Institute at www.tmc.edu/thi/cooley.html and www.wic.org/bio/debakey.htm

Jacob (Jack) Kolff's memories of growing up in wartime Holland and later of working with his father on artificial heart development were published in *Artificial Organs*, the journal of the American Society for Artificial Internal Organs, vol. 22, no. 11 (1998)

The Kingdom of the Netherlands in World War II, by L. de Jong

The Patients, by Jurgen Thorwald (Droemer Knaur Verlag Schoeller & Co., Zurich, published in 1971 and available in English translation), contains interviews with now deceased assistants working in Kampen at the time of the early experiments, and an interview with Sofia Schafstadt.

The website of the International Society of Nephrology contains interviews with pioneers in this field, including Kolff, and a comprehensive bibliography of the history of nephrology compiled by Professor J. Stewart Cameron at http://www.isn-online.org/

INDEX

Note: Willem Kolff is abreviated to WK. Major entries are in chronological order, where appropriate.

Abbott Laboratories 147
Abel, John Jacob 39, 40, 41, 67
Acme Company, Cleveland 141
Akutsu, Dr Ted 144, 153
albumen in blood 14, 80
Alkmaar 30
allergic reactions 39
Allis-Chalmers kidney 134
Alwall, Nils 119, 157
America see USA
American Medical Association 137
American Society of Artificial Internal Organs 162
Amsterdam 46, 90–1, 92–3, 110–11
animals
  experiments on see cows; dogs
  WK's love of 25–6
anti-coagulants see heparin; hirudin
Apeldoorn 57, 102
apparatus 66

arm, artificial 158
Arnhem 64, 103
arteries 96
'Ausweiss' (medical exemption certificate) 57–8
autopsies 31
awards 48, 121, 124, 172, 173, 181–2

Baatz (German commander) 105–8
babies, operations on 139–40, 141–2
Bailey, Dr Charles 136–7, 151
Barnard, Christiaan 173
Baxter Travenol 148
Baylor University 162
Beekbergen 22–5, 102
Berk, Hendrik 68, 69, 72, 88, 99
Best, Charles Herbert 44
Bjork, Viking Olov 126–7
blood
  analysis 58
  cells 63, 70, 94, 136, 166

circulation 35–6
clotting 39, 43–4, 161, 167
    see also heparin
groups 47
plasma 47
pressure 6, 38, 81, 115
protiens 127
transfusions 49, 92
vessels 96
blood banks 46–8, 89
Boele, Gustav 78–80
Boerhaave, Herman 19–20
Borne, Kreutz Wendedich von
    dem 50
Borst, Prof 128
Brandenburger, Jacques E.
    41–2
Brinkman, Prof Robert 40,
    62–3, 67, 123
Bruning, Jan 38, 41, 116
budgets 70–1, 75
Bundle of His 142
burette 83, 84
Bywaters, Dr Eric 118

cadavers, experiments with
    125–6
calcium 5
calves, experiments on 161,
    164–5, 169
Canada 118, 119
canulas 85, 126
carpentry, WK's love of 23–4,
    36, 88, 121

Carroll, Diana 178
cellophane 11, 40–2, 76, 147
    in oxygenators 127
    sterilising 82–3
    see also sausage skin
cellulose 39, 41, 146
cephalin 43
Christiansen, Gen 91
chronic nephritis 81
Clark, Barney 164–8
Cleef, Greta 93–5
Cleveland Clinic, Ohio 130,
    132–3, 140–3, 150–2,
    155
collaborators see Nazi
    sympathisers
collodion 39, 40
Columbia Presbyterian
    Hospital, New York 47
Cooley, Denton 138, 162–3,
    165
County Cook Hospital,
    Chicago 47
cows/calves, experiments on
    127–8, 136, 161,
    164–5, 169
creatinine 85
cytoscopy 114

Daniels, Prof Polak 35–6, 38,
    50
DeBakey, Michael 162–3
DeVries, William 163, 164,
    166, 170

diagnostic methods 122–3,
132
dialysers *see* kidney machines
dialysing fluid 39, 41, 67, 68,
73, 79, 149
dialysis 13–15, 76–8, 87,
89–90, 96, 178
early failures listed 98–9
electrolyte equilibrium in
76–7
first continuous 83–6
first successful 115–16,
117–18
abroad 118–19
swelling reduced during 93
Dijk, E.C. van 68, 69
Division of Artificial Organs
158–9
Dobelle, William 175, 176
dogs, experiments on 39, 78,
134, 138–9, 153
Domingo (engineer) 57–8
Drew, Dr Charles 47

ear, artificial 158, 175
Effler, Dr 139
Eindhoven 92
electrolytes 76, 85, 94–5, 115
Engelberg 146
engineers, work with 57–8,
134, 143, 155, 158–9
Episcopal Hospital,
Philadelphia 137
Eskes, Willy 75, 84, 115, 179

eye
artificial 1, 158, 175, 176
damage to 38, 81

feudal system 18–19, 28–9
First World War 22, 39, 44
fistula 4
flame photometer 57–8
Food & Drugs Administration
(FDA) 169
Friesland 36–8
fundraising *see* sponsorship

Gardner, W.James 135
Gastman, Revd 82
Germany, plastics manufacture
in 168–9
Gibbon, Dr John 137–8
glomeruli 6, 90
glucose 47, 94–5
Groningen 30, 32, 34–6, 38,
49–51, 62, 80, 102
Gronstein, Paul Lester 5–6

Haas, Georg 39
haemoglobin 47
haemolysis 70
Hague, The 44, 49, 89, 90,
117
Hammersmith Hospital,
London 118
Harken, Dr Dwight 137
heart
anti-coagulant damages 39

artificial 1, 125, 134, 153–4,
    158, 159–65, 177
    cost reductions in 168–9
    opposition to 160
    problems 161–2, 164,
        166, 167–8
    types 159–60
    described 160–1
    surgery 136–40
heart/lung machine 134,
    135–43, 158, 166
heparin 11, 13, 40, 42–3, 77,
    79
    discovery of 43–4
    dosage increased 85
hirudin 39
Hitler, Adolf 50, 91, 128
Holmer, Dr 90
Holzenbein, Dr 148
Hotel Rijnland 21
Howell, William H. 43
Hummelo 21–2
Hursic, Larry 141
hypertension 130, 133, 145

Ijssel river 53, 64, 102, 104, 111
illnesses, symptoms faked 57–9
income 70–1, 131, 155
infants, operations on 139–40,
    141–2
infection 98
insulin 39, 43, 44, 105
intra-aortic balloon pump
    152–3

Jacobsen, Steve 153
Jacobze, Dr John 173
Jarvik, Robert 159–60, 165–6,
    169, 170
jaundice 58, 114
Jews 9, 50, 56, 60, 72, 78–9,
    104
    killed 106
John Hopkins University,
    Baltimore 176
Jones, David 170
journals, medical 72, 119–20
juice can dialyser 146–8

Kampen 31, 52–3, 123, 136
    described 52–3
    people described 53–4
    wartime 67–8, 88, 92, 100,
        103, 109
        conscripted workers in
            104–6
        liberation 110–12
Kampen Enamel Works 68–71,
    88, 95
Kampen Hospital 9–16, 61–4,
    171, 179
    laboratory in 62, 74–5,
        124–5
    Room 12a 10, 14, 114–16,
        171–2, 174
    wartime 12, 72, 100, 103,
        106–7
    postwar 113–16, 129,
        173–4

Karp, Haskell 163
Kehrer, Dr 66, 105, 113–14
kidney
  failure described 38
  function described 5–6,
    12–13
  transplant 6–7, 150–2
kidney, artificial 158, 170
  Allis-Chalmers 134
  attitudes to 66–7, 89, 96,
    114–15, 128, 135
  disposable 145–7
  first successful 11–16, 68–74
    payment for 70–1
  juice can dialyser 146–8
  Kolff/Brigham 123–4
  methods of construction
    72–4, 88–9
  nose-cone dialyser 149–50
  problems with 68–70, 71,
    76–8
    blood cell damage 78, 94
    clotting 77–8
    continuous motion 67,
      69–70, 149
    electrolyte imbalance
      76–7
    quantities of blood 42
    surface area 41, 42–3, 67,
      68–9
  reputation of 119
  rotating drum 133
  transport of 91, 92, 118
  twin-coil dialyser 146–8

  washing machine type 3–4,
    149
  wearable 153
  wind-it-yourself dialyser
    148–9, 158
kiewiet (lapwing) eggs 121–2
Klinkmann, Dr Horst 157–8,
  168, 174
Koch, Robert 24
Kolff, Adrie (daughter)
  born 53, 112, 121–2
  in USA 129–31, 144–5
Kolff, Cornelius (grandfather)
  17–18, 19
Kolff, Cornelius 'Kees' (son)
  111
Kolff, Jack (son) 34, 45, 55,
  121, 124–5, 176
  emigrates to USA 129–31
  as heart surgeon 163–4,
    166, 169
  observations on WK 132–3,
    146
Kolff, Jacob (father) 2, 19–23,
  24
Kolff, Janke (née Huidekoper,
  wife) 27–8, 79–80,
  129, 156
  engagement & marriage
    27–8, 30, 32, 33–4,
    143–5
  separation 178
  in wartime 61, 111–12
  emigration 123, 131

inheritance 29, 71, 131
Kolff, Kees (brother) 23
Kolff, Mimi (aunt) 130, 132
Kolff, Mrs (mother) 20–1, 22
Kolff, Therus (son) 129
Kolff, Willem Johan 'Pim'
      (b.1911) pp181–2
   appearance 9
   birth & childhood 18,
      21–7
   student 28–34, 50
   family life 33–4, 121–2
   and Nazis, negotiating with
      105–9
   emigrates to USA 129–30
   in retirement 171–9
   character
      bravery 108–9
      compassion 26
      empathy 75
      kindness 64
      politeness 64
      willingness to admit
         failure 80
   originality of ideas 30–1,
      71–2, 124, 141, 176
   problem-solving 67, 71,
      146
   published work 31–2, 72,
      110, 116–17, 118, 122,
      158–9
   statue described 172
   legacy 175–6
Kolff Associates 165, 169

Kolff Institute 172–3
Kolff/Brigham kidney 123–4
Kollf, Albert (son) 100
Krakow 118
Krüseman (Janke's
      grandfather) 46, 71

laboratories 170
   described 62, 74–5, 124–5,
      134–5, 156
   fire destroys 159
Landsteiner, Karl 47
lapwing eggs 121–2
lectures 122, 123, 128, 174,
      176–8
leeches 39
Leeuw, Nannie van de 63–4,
      118–19
Lehrke (German commander)
      108
Leiden
   cattle market 21
   University 19–20, 25,
      26–32, 128
Leij, Mieneke van der 62, 74,
      84, 116, 179
Leningrad 47
Limberg 92, 103
limbs, artificial 158
Liotta, Domingo 163
Liotta heart 162
lung
   anti-coagulant damages 39
   artificial 178–9

McLean, Jay 43

Maytag washing machine 149

medical establishment 132,
151, 152

medical journals 72, 119–20

Merrill, John 150–1

Michael, Prof 49

Middelharnis 17

milking machine 127, 141

mitral commissurotomy 136–7

money 29, 34, 70–1, 75, 131
commercial value of
inventions 143, 174
payments for operations 86,
163
sponsorship/fundraising
122, 156, 158, 169

motor 74, 79–80

Moulopoulis, Spyros 152

Mount Sinai Hospital,
Cleveland 158

Mount Sinai Hospital, New
York 118, 122, 124

Murray, Joseph 119–20,
123–4

Mycosis Fungoides 31–2

NASA 149–50

National Socialists *see* Nazi
sympathisers

Nazi sympathisers 15, 50, 59,
60–1, 68, 106, 171
assassination attempts 64–5,
101

Kolff's attitude to 15–16
treatment of after war 113,
117

Nazis, WK's negotiations with
105–9

nephritis 81, 90, 93

New York 118, 122, 123, 124

newspapers 165–6, 168

Nijmegen 63, 64

Nobel Prize 124, 174

Noordweg 33–4

Noordwijk, Jacob 'Bob' van
51, 75, 80, 83–6,
89–93, 97
background 62–3
in hiding 100–3
after war 119, 173, 176,
179

nose-cone dialyser 149–50

oedema 94

Olmstead, Rick 134, 143

open-heart surgery 137–40

Operation Market Garden
102–3

Oppasser (manservant) 29

Oudshoorn, Commandant
113, 117

over-hydration 167

Overflakkee 17

oxygenator 124–8, 136, 170
bubble 167
disc 126–7
membrane 139, 140–1, 166

problems with 140–2
screen 137–8

pacemakers 142–3
Page, Irvine 130, 133–4, 135, 142–3, 145–6
patents 143, 148, 161
pathology 31
Pel, Dr 104
Peter Bent Brigham Hospital, Boston 123, 124, 150
picric acid 58
Poland 118
polio virus 43
polyethylene 138
polyurethane 161
Post (farmer) 60–1
potassium salts 5, 58, 74, 76, 114, 115
Poutos, Gene 151–2
press 165–6, 168
pressure cooker 146
prostate gland 78
protocol for operations 140
Public Health Service 158
published works 31–2, 72, 110, 116–18, 122, 147, 158–9
pumps 70, 71–2, 126, 136
for artificial heart 162
intra-aortic balloon 152–3
roller 141–2

quinine 29, 34

rations 56, 57, 70, 91, 110–11
Red Cross 46, 49, 91, 105, 107
research
assistants 156–7
obstacles to 142–3
sponsorship/fundraising 122, 156, 158, 169
resistance 55–61, 64, 113
Room 12a 10, 14, 114–16, 171–2, 174
Rotterdam 21, 44–5, 48–9, 103–4, 108, 111
Rowntree, Leonard 39, 40, 67
Royal Victoria Hospital, Montreal 118
Russia 91, 128

St John's Hospital, Baltimore 43
saline solution 39, 68
Salt Lake City 155–6, 170, 174
Sandberg, Mayor 106–7, 108
sausage skin 11, 12, 13, 42, 66–70, 87
fragility of 14, 71, 79, 84, 96
see also cellophane
Schafstadt, Sofia 10–16, 113–17, 128
Schoot, Abraham van der 106
Schrijver, Janny 81–7, 89
Scribner, Belding 150
Second World War 12, 44–51, 100–1, 104

German occupation 54–61, 70, 72, 88, 91–2
    conscription of labour 91–2, 102, 103–6
    preparations for 36
    surrender of Holland 45
    end of 9–10, 111–12
sewing-machine motor 74, 79–80
Siegfried Line 102
Sierat, Jan 29
Snapper, Prof Isador 122–3, 129, 132
Soames, Dr 139
sodium salts 5, 47, 76
Spaander, Dr 92
sponsorship/fundraising 122, 156, 158, 169
Starling's Law 162
sterilisation procedures 82–3, 91
streptomycin 24, 124
strikes of Dutch workers 92
sulphonamide 114
Sweden 127
Sybrandaburen 36–8

telephone network 57
Tendeloo, Prof 30–1
Termeulen (patient) 97–8
Thalimer 41
theophylline 167
Thorn, Dr George 123
thrombin (enzyme) 43

tin cans 146–7
Topaz, Stephen 152, 170
Toronto 119
toxins 12–13, 14, 38, 69, 81, 116
tuberculosis 50
    renal 89
    sanitorium 22–5, 102
    symptoms faked 59
Turnbull, Rupert 133
Turner, B.B. 39, 40, 67

'Uncle Joe' 58–9
University Hospital, Salt Lake City 165
uraemia 6, 81, 85
    paper on 72–4
urea 67, 69, 85, 90, 97–8
    crystals 6, 38, 97
    early attempts to remove 38–9
    levels in blood 13–14, 42, 81, 86, 93, 114, 115
uric acid 85
urine 5, 47, 89, 95, 98, 114, 116
USA 122–4, 129–33
    differences in methodology 132
    early experiments in 39, 43
    WK emigrates to 129–31
Utah, University of 155–7, 158, 161, 174
Utrecht 45, 128, 173

vacuum forming 168–9
veins 96, 126
visas, WK arranges 157–8
vitamin D 43

Walter, Carl 123–4
Warner, Dr Homer 155
washing machine 3, 149
Watschinger, Dr Bruno 145–7
webbing 148

Welle, Sister M. ter 115
West, Pop van 26–7
Winchell, Dr Paul 161
wood, WK's love of 23–4, 36, 88, 121
World Health Organisation (WHO) 146

zoos 25–6
Zwolle 52, 81, 127